The Practical Treatment of
BACKACHE
—and—
SCIATICA

Other books by D.N. Golding

Synopsis of Rheumatic Diseases. 4th edn., John Wright, 1982

Concise Management of the Common Rheumatic Disorders, John Wright, 1979

Tutorials in Rheumatology, Pitman Medical, 1980

Problems in Arthritis and Rheumatism, MTP Press, 1981

The Practical Treatment of
BACKACHE
—and—
SCIATICA

John Barrett, MB, DPhys Med, MRO
Orthopaedic Physician and Clinical Assistant in Rheumatology
Princess Alexandra Hospital, Harlow, Essex

and

Douglas N. Golding MA, MD, FRCPI
Consultant Rheumatologist, West Essex Health Authority

Director, Rheumatology Unit, West Essex Health Authority
Princess Alexandra Hospital, Harlow, Essex

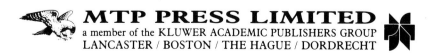
MTP PRESS LIMITED
a member of the KLUWER ACADEMIC PUBLISHERS GROUP
LANCASTER / BOSTON / THE HAGUE / DORDRECHT

Published in the UK and Europe by
MTP Press Limited
Falcon House
Lancaster, England

British Library Cataloguing in Publication Data

Barrett, John
   The practical treatment of backache and sciatica.
   1.   Backache.
   I.   Title   II. Golding, Douglas N.
   616.7′306   RD768

ISBN 0-85200-773-6

Published in the USA by
MTP Press
A division of Kluwer Boston Inc
190 Old Derby Street
Hingham, MA 02043, USA

Library of Congress Cataloging in Publication Data

Barrett, John, 1930–
   The practical treatment of backache and sciatica.

   Bibliography: p.
   Includes Index
   1.   Backache–Treatment.   2.   Sciatica–Treatment.
   I.   Golding, Douglas Noel.   II.   Title   [DNLM:
   1.   Backache–Therapy.   2.   Sciatica–Therapy.   WE 720 B274p]
   RD768.B37   1984   617′.56   84–3872

ISBN 0-85200-773-6

Printed in Great Britain by
Redwood Burn Limited, Trowbridge

Contents

Preface

Backache is one of the most common ailments of the human race. Although a distressing condition and a frequent cause of absence from work – it is said that eighteen million working days are lost per year because of back pain – it is amazing how neglected has been the study of its cause and treatment, at least until relatively recent years. This may be reflected in the rarity of photographs of the posterior view of Venus de Milo, as compared with the well-known view from the front! (Figure 1). Undergraduate teaching of backache is scanty, partly because backache is not considered very important as it is rarely due to 'serious' disease and recovery is often spontaneous. However, this is not always the case and a significant number of patients have recurrences and fail to respond to conventional treatment.

There are many possible causes of backache and physicians and orthopaedic surgeons continue to disagree as to which are the most

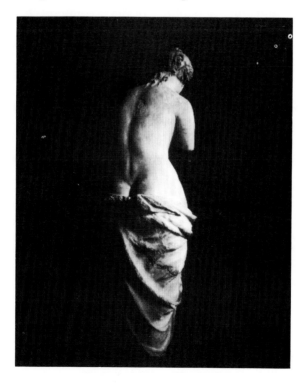

Figure 1 The Venus de Milo

important factors and hence the best treatment. Proper scientific treatment must await deeper knowledge of the aetiology and pathology; meanwhile, management will have to be empirical, at least to some extent. Nevertheless, there is a strong case for establishing guidelines for treatment. Many physicians feel helpless about the best way to handle an individual patient with backache. Should bed rest be advocated, or should the opposite line be taken – should the spine be mobilized? Analgesics are obviously needed – but are anti-inflammatory agents helpful? Is it a disservice to the patient not to request specialist advice?

In this book, backache is presented as a variety of 'syndromes' based principally on clinical and to some extent radiological features. The pattern of treatment will largely depend on the type of syndrome and its severity and chronicity. This classification is based on the assumption that backache is most often due to either an intervertebral disc lesion, spondylosis or osteoarthritis of the spine, or one or more intervertebral (facet) joint derangements. Symptoms may be due to a combination of these, but in all cases it is the *syndrome* rather than the exact lesion on which the principles of treatment are based, always keeping in mind the possibility of less common but important conditions, such as ankylosing spondylitis and bone tumours.

One of the best current books on back pain is *The Lumbar Spine and Back Pain* (edited by M. Jayson), in which only three of 17 chapters are devoted to treatment. A much more treatment-orientated approach is adopted by the present book, which may be regarded as the logical successor to a recent book by Dr David P. Evans entitled *Backache – Its Evolution and Conservative Treatment* (also published by MTP Press Ltd). *The Practical Treatment of Backache and Sciatica* is entirely devoted to management from the practical point of view, being the result of the combined views of a rheumatologist and an osteopathic physician. Basic theory is mentioned where relevant, but it is always practical aspects of treatment which are emphasized. Therefore, while the book is principally aimed towards general practitioner readership, it is hoped that rheumatologists, orthopaedic surgeons and those in training may also find it useful.

J. Barrett
D.N. Golding

References

Jayson, M. (ed.) (1980). *The Lumbar Spine and Back Pain*. 2nd Edn. (London: Pitman Medical)

Evans, D.P. (1982). *Backache – Its Evolution and Conservative Treatment*. (Lancaster: MTP Press)

Foreword

The well trodden paths to the doors of osteopaths, chiropracters and acupuncturists, bear eloquent testimony to the frequency of backache and the inadequacy of its treatment by most clinicians. The naive suggestion that this commonest of all rheumatic syndromes is due to man's upright posture has long since been exploded. Numerous quadrepeds have disc problems of even greater severity than bipedal man. In many sufferers the circuitory of their frontal lobes may be of more significance than their spinal posture. This may explain some of the success of unorthodox practitioners, in that at least they listen to the patient. One friend of mine with acute lumbago said that the surgeon to whom he was referred paid as much attention to him as the Queen does to her subjects as she passes down the Mall – a gracious, although necessarily, perfunctory, acknowledgement.

We are grateful to organisations like the Arthritis and Rheumatism Council and the Back Pain Research Association for promoting clinical and fundamental research into this morass of conditions. A greater understanding of patho-physiology is of the utmost importance, although it does not guarantee a cure. Patients are only mildly interested in the fundamentals. They wish to feel better and return to work. The present employment situation has made the latter consideration even more pressing. A prospective study we were undertaking in general practice with Dr Max Roberts and Dr Sam Ofei on the merits of bed rest, lumbo-sacral supports given immediately and strong analgesia on its own, was ruined by the present government's economic policies – the stream of possible patients dried up at source. General practitioners, rheumatologists and orthopaedic surgeons share the patients concern for help. A handy volume of 100 pages length that serves as a 'cook book' on backache and sciatica would be most welcome. Here we have it!

V. Wright
Professor
of Rheumatology
University of Leeds

1
Introduction

1. WHAT MAKES A BACK ACHE?

There are many causes of backache, but the commonest conditions are intervertebral disc lesions, intervertebral (facet) joint derangements and spondylosis or osteoarthritis. Clinical examination often suggests the lesion, X-rays are less often helpful and indeed are often misleading – for example, showing degenerative changes in the spine which may have little or no bearing on the cause of the pain. Myelography may be more helpful, but only in certain situations such as frank disc prolapses with root involvement. We can confirm a peptic ulcer by carrying out gastroscopy or lung cancer by bronchoscopy, but only surgical exploration will provide absolute proof that nerve root pressure is due to a prolapsed disc.

While the conditions mentioned are undoubtedly responsible for the great majority of backache seen in practice, one must never exclude the possibility of important, if less common, conditions such as ankylosing spondylitis, metabolic bone disease, bone tumours and others. How to investigate conditions such as these is described later in this chapter.

It should be mentioned that some maintain that involvement of the dura mater or its root sleeve, i.e. its prolongation around an emerging nerve root, by a disc protrusion is the usual factor responsible for back pain, with or without sciatica, and that the lumbar intervertebral joints are insensitive to internal derangement – that is to deny the existence of the deranged intervertebral joint 'facet syndrome' (on which osteopathic practice is based). This would imply that the success of manipulation is entirely dependent on reducing a disc prolapse thereby relieving pressure on the dura. It is more widely

1

believed, however, that a disc prolapse should not be diagnosed unless there is clear objective evidence of lumbar nerve-root pressure as shown by reflex changes or other neurological signs in the legs. However, it is generally felt that limitation of straight-leg-raising, a cardinal sign of lower lumbar disc lesions, is really a manifestation of dural irritation, the degree of limitation relating to the size of the disc prolapse. This has important connotations regarding treatment: for example, that an epidural injection is less likely to be effective in patients with a 'large' disc prolapse, generally speaking where straight-leg-raising is less than 45° (see Chapter 8).

Degenerative conditions of the discs and vertebrae are often lumped under the heading 'osteoarthritis' or 'spondylosis'. In fact these are anatomically, pathologically and clinically different conditions. *Spondylosis* (or anterior spondylosis) implies disc degeneration with consequent reactive osteophytosis, radiologically described as lipping. The term *osteoarthritis* should be confined to involvement of the facet (intervertebral) joints, which are true synovial joints and therefore undergo true osteoarthritis. Spondylosis is often amenable to simple therapy, except where there is associated vertebral instability (spondylolisthesis) which can be problematical. On the other hand, facet-joint osteoarthritis can be resistant to treatment – particularly in overweight, lordotic patients who often have generalized osteoarthritis. In this condition, as in peripheral osteoarthritis, acute inflammatory flare-ups of backache may occur. Incidentally, these synovial joints can also be involved by gout or pseudo-gout (chondrocalcinosis) and local deposition of calcium apatite or pyrophosphate crystals, sometimes seen in the X-ray, may be associated with acute localized pain.

What receptors for pain exist in the spine and surrounding structures? Theoretically, pain can arise in nociceptive receptors of several tissues, including apophyseal joint capsules, ligaments, periosteum, dura and epidural fibroadipose tissue. There are no nociceptive receptors in the intervertebral disc. Root pain results from the intervertebral disc impinging on the nociceptive nervous plexuses of the dural root sleeves, both mechanically and also resulting from inflammatory changes which follow an acute prolapse.

2. ANATOMICAL AND PATHOLOGICAL FACTS

We should say something of the intervertebral discs and the intervertebral (apophyseal or facet) joints if we are to assume that the majority of back pain arises from these. We shall also briefly mention the spinal ligaments and paravertebral muscles.

Spinal ligaments

These are the posterior longitudinal ligament (mainly attached to the discs), the ligamentous flavum (joining the laminae) and the inter-spinous ligaments (joining the spinous processes).

Intervertebral discs

These consist of the outer cartilaginous plates, the annulus fibrosus composed (of fibrous tissue) and the nucleus pulposus (composed of gelatinous tissue). The discs are avascular. They lose fluid and become fibrous, less elastic and narrower with age. The nucleus pulposus can be regarded as a ballbearing, with the vertebral bodies rolling over the incompressible gel while the posterior intervertebral joints guide and steady the movement. The nucleus does not contain sensory nerves, these being contained in the annulus fibrosus and longitudinal ligaments. In general, herniation of the nucleus pulposus through a split in the annulus is due to a combination of the latter and trauma. Herniation is either (a) posterolateral, the nucleus displacing the posterior longitudinal ligament to one side and compressing emerging nerveroots and sciatica or (b) posterior ('central') causing back pain only. (Very rarely there is spinal cord compression and myelopathy in a central disc prolapse).

Spinal muscles

The erector spinae, extending from the neck to the sacrum, has three layers: superficial (the most powerful), intermediate and deep. These are spinal extensors – the rectus abdominas and other abdominal muscles are the flexors. They are secondary causes of back pain, mainly as a result of reflex hyperactivity (muscle spasm).

The segmental innervation of the principal muscles involved by root lesion is as follows:

Hip flexion	$L_{2,3}$	Hip extension	$L_{4,5}$
Knee flexion	L_5, S_1	Knee extension	$L_{3,4}$
Ankle dorsiflexion	$L_{4,5}$	Ankle plantar flexion	$S_{1,2}$
Foot inversion	L_4	Foot eversion	L_5, S_1

Spinal dermatomes

These are depicted in Figure 2.

Transitional lumbar vertebrae

A transitional lumbar vertebra is said to occur when there is sacral-

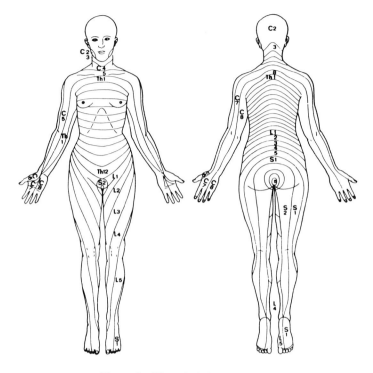

Figure 2 The spinal dermatomes

ization of the first sacral segment. This is said to have no clinical significance, but some feel that this congenital anomaly predisposes to adjacent disc degeneration. More specifically, unilateral sacralization of L_5, where there is often pseudarthrosis (false joint formation) between the transverse process and the ala of the sacrum, may give rise to low back pain because the pivotal axis of the lumbo-sacral joint is transferred from the central position to the pseudarthrosis.

Lumbar spinal canal

The spinal cord extends to the L_1/L_2 junction. It is bounded as shown in Figure 3.

Spinal stenosis, i.e. narrowing of the spinal canal, can be congenital or acquired – usually by spondylosis, occasionally spondylolisthesis. The spinal canal can be oval, triangular, deltoid or trefoil.

The trefoil canal is especially associated with spinal stenosis – the lateral recesses are very shallow and fully occupied by the nerve roots,

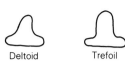

Deltoid   Trefoil

so that any further intrusion into this space (as by spondylosis) will compress the roots. Spinal flexion increases the size of the canal so relieving symptoms (see also Chapter 11.3).

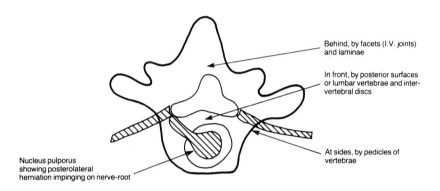

Behind, by facets (I.V. joints) and laminae

In front, by posterior surfaces or lumbar vertebrae and intervertebral discs

At sides, by pedicles of vertebrae

Nucleus pulporus showing posterolateral herniation impinging on nerve-root

Figure 3   Anterior view of a lumber spinal vertebra

Intervertebral (apophyseal or facet) joints

These are the joints between the superior and inferior articular processes; their importance has already been stressed. These synovial joints can become inflamed and thus painful, as mentioned above. They are frequently the cause of episodes of back pain as a result of minor slips, called facet lesions or intervertebral joint derangements. They can be involved with microfractures (fatigue fractures) and tiny loose bodies can even form within the joints. Nerve root pressure may result from osteophytes projecting into the intervertebral foramina from the margins of osteoarthritic apophyseal joints, but more often pain may be referred into the groins or legs, without evidence of objective nerve root pressure.

Intervertebral foraminae

The nerve roots emerge through these foraminae. They are bounded

5

in front by the posterior surface of the vertebral body and disc, behind by the apophyseal (facet) joint, above by the inferior surface of the vertebra and below by the pedicle.

Vertebral instability

This is an important concept in the pathogenesis of back pain. Spinal hypermobility (see Chapter 2.1) predisposes to this. In its more severe forms, spondylolisthesis may occur. Otherwise minor degrees of vertebral instability often account for or aggravate back pain which is resistant to mobilization or traction, and requires stabilization by a corset, isometric exercises or sometimes sclerosing injections (see Chapter 6).

Spondylolisthesis

Slipping forward (spondylolisthesis) or backward (retro-spondylolisthesis) of one vertebra on the other is due to instability because of either (a) a congenital lesion of the pars interarticularis of the apophyseal joint (spondylolysis), (b) a stress fracture of the pars or (c) secondary to osteoarthritis of the apophyseal joints. In congenital lesions and stress fractures the deficiency in the pars interarticularis (in radiological parlance, the neural arch) can be seen in oblique views, while this is not so in osteoarthritis. Stress fractures in this situation, which develop early in life, do not show the typical excessive callus formation normally seen. Spondylolisthesis occassionally causes back pain in young persons, but usually not until associated degenerative changes start at 35–45 years and especially so in later life when osteoarthritis of the facet joints due to the resulting incongruity has become established. Spondylolysis and spondylolisthesis are further considered in Chapter 12.2.

Sacro-iliac joints

Argument still rages as to whether any significant movement takes place at the sacro-iliac joints. However, though there is now considerable evidence that this is the case and that 'sacro-iliac strain' (beloved by osteopaths) can sometimes occur, this is not a common cause of backache. There is little doubt that most pain felt over the sacro-iliac joint is referred from the spine. Sacro-iliac strain pain is commoner in women, especially during and after pregnancy. Of course, there is no argument that pain does arise directly from the sacro-iliac joints when these are inflamed, as in sacro-iliitis and ankylosing spondylitis.

3. HOW TO EXAMINE THE SPINE

Taking the history

The physician's first task is to distinguish patients with common *mechanical problems* of the back (such as disc lesions and ligamentous strains) from those with more serious *pathological lesions* (such as bone tumours and ankylosing spondylitis and those with *pronounced psychological factors*. A careful history, with time spent listening to the patient's account of how his symptoms developed, is important.

As will be explained in Chapter 2, the common backache syndromes are those due to intervertebral joint derangements, prolapsed discs, chronic osteoarthritis of the spine and ligamentous postural backache.

The typical *disc syndrome* starts as a central low back pain which after a few days becomes unilateral and spreads down to the buttock and leg. Relief of backache and stiffness with the onset of sciatica is pathognomonic of disc herniation. It is widely known that radicular pain is often intensified by coughing but, as many patients do not cough, a useful alternative question is: 'Does it increase the pain when you strain at stool?'

The patient with an *acute intervertebral joint derangement* giving a typical attack of lumbago has often experienced similar attacks before and, as they usually follow the same pattern, listening to their account supplies a ready-made diagnosis and prognosis for the present episode.

As regards the much less common '*pathological backache*', if questioned directly patients often admit to malaise or other features of general ill health. Gradually increasing pain (especially if unrelenting at night) calls for further investigation.

With regard to *psychogenic backache*, it is always better to ask every patient about their mental state (has anything happened to cause increased tension, anxiety or depression?) when taking the history, rather than find nothing wrong on examination and then introduce the subject – when the patient, not unreasonably, often thinks he has been written off as 'neurotic'. The grossly neurotic patient is usually vague about the onset and distribution of pain and paraesthesiae, being much more concerned with general dissatisfaction over his lot, his doctors and all his previous treatment.

Summarizing history taking in back pain and sciatica, the following are important:

7

(1) History of injury to the back

(2) Pain   situation and spread
             increase with coughing or straining at stool
             whether worse at night

(3) Segmental paraesthesiae in one or both legs

(4) Mental state

(5) Morning stiffness (especially important in ankylosing
     spondylitis)

(6) Bowel and bladder function

(7) Stress and occupational factors

(8) Family history of back trouble

The examination

The spine is first examined standing, then lying on the back (supine)
and finally lying on the stomach (prone).

(a) *Examination standing*

Inspection of the patient standing will show gross postural faults, such
as thoracic kyphosis perhaps developing as a result of previous
Scheuermann's disease (osteochondritis) or a pelvic shift to one side
with lumbar muscle spasm indicating a disc lesion. In young patients
with postural backache it is important to see whether there is any
marked difference in leg lengths. This can be assessed by asking the
patient to bend forward and taking a sight along the spine, when a
short leg will show as a falling away of the buttock on that side (see
Figure 4). This can be confirmed by an erect X-ray of the pelvis
showing the upper ends of the femora. The feet should also be in-
spected, to see if they collapse into planus on standing – flat feet often
put a strain on the back (see Chapter 8.1).

Next the *movements of the lumbar spine* are tested. The patient is asked
to forward bend, backward bend and side-bend to each side and a
note is made if all or some of these movements are restricted or painful. 'Blocking' of one movement, the rest being free, strongly suggests a
mechanical derangement of one of the spinal intervertebral joints. A
painful arc of movement on flexion with deviation to one side is
indicative of a small disc lesion. While the patient is standing it is a
useful moment to test the power of the plantar-flexors and dorsiflexors
of the ankle. The patient is asked to stand on tiptoe (ankle plantar-

flexion), testing the calf muscles suppled by L_5. If the patient can bend down to put his hands flat on the ground, this suggests a hyper-mobile ('loose') back which may or may not be part of a general hypermobility syndrome, and other joints should be tested for hypermobility.

(b) *Examination supine*

With the patient supine, the *straight-leg-raising* test (SLR) is most important. A note is made of the angle at which pain commences and the level to which the leg can be comfortably taken before reflex muscle spasm prevents further raising. Occasionally one meets a 'crossed positive SLR', where raising the apparently good leg pro-duces pain on the opposite side; this occurs in a paracaudal disc

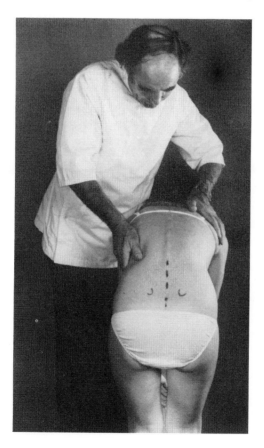

Figure 4   Siting along the spine to detect the falling away of one buttock indicating a short leg

9

protrusion, where raising the good leg pulls the affected nerve root more centrally and hence produces pain in it.

Next the *knee reflexes* are tested and the power in the quadriceps and hamstring muscles. There is no need to test sensation if the patient does not complain of pins and needles or numbness, but if so it is important to define the area of objective numbness. First light touch and then pinprick appreciation is tested.

The *ankle-jerks* can also be tested while the patient lies supine, but less readily than when prone – a doubtful ankle-jerk elicited in the supine position will often become more evident when tested in the prone position. Finally, the brief neurological examination is completed by eliciting the plantar responses.

Next the *sacro-iliac tests* are performed. These are 'gapping' and compression of the pelvis (sacro-iliac springing) with the examiner's hands on the anterior iliac spines (Figure 5). The patient is asked to disregard pain at the front and note any pain over the sacro-iliac joints at the back, especially if this is more marked on one side. It is comparatively uncommon for gapping or other sacro-iliac tests to produce pain from mechanical strains of the sacro-iliac joint and, while these tests are never definitive of sacro-iliitis, if positive it is always worth having these joints X-rayed.

Next the *hip joints* can be examined for restriction of movements, but

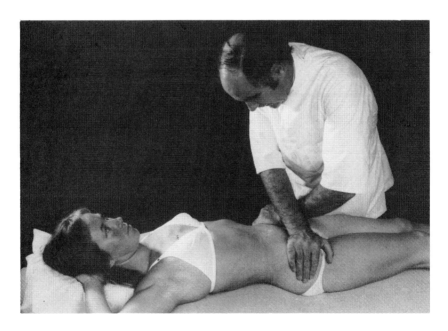

Figure 5   Sacro-iliac gapping test

it should be pointed out that in sciatica and in lumbar lesions some limitation or pain on hip-joint movements is often found because at the extremes of movement the spinal joints or nerve roots may be put in tension. Alternatively, some degree of capsular contraction occurs in upper lumbar lesions giving a false impression of osteoarthritis of the hips. At this stage it is also essential to *palpate the abdomen* and this is a good opportunity to ask the patient whether he or she has any trouble with passing water or has noticed any numbness in the perineum, if this has not already come out in the history. Next the *peripheral pulses* are assessed at the femoral level and at the ankle, where either the posterior tibial or the dorsalis pedis pulses should be palpable. Should there be any suspicion of pelvic pathology, *rectal and pelvic examinations* should be carried out, though these are not routinely required.

(c) *Examination side-lying*

Next the patient is turned onto his side and, with the knees flexed up, using a rocking movement of the spine individual movements of the lumbar joints are palpated (Figure 6). Here one tries to assess whether one segment of the lumbar spine is particularly stiff, or whether there is general hypermobility (as in the loose back) due to

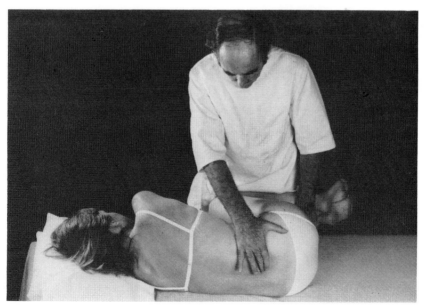

Figure 6 The individual movements of the lumbar joints are palpated in the side-lying position

lax ligaments. It is also often possible to get the first clue to spondyl-olisthesis by this examination: a 'shelf' at the spinous processes will be apparent and there is hypermobility at the segment above (Figure 7a). For example, in spondylolisthesis of L_5 on the sacrum, the shelf and hypermobility are felt at the L_{4-5} level, because the spinous process of L_5 is left behind in the slip (Figure 7b).

(d) *Examination prone (lying on the abdomen)*

With the patient lying prone on the examination couch the lumbar spine is tested by 'springing' with the palm of the hand. Starting at the sacrum each segment is 'sprung' in turn and a note is made of muscle guarding or pain (Figure 8). This is also useful to elicit pain in the sacro-iliac joints in sacro-iliitis and in alerting one to the possibility of pathological conditions if there is marked muscle guard-ing, especially in the lower thoracic or upper lumbar spine where mechanical conditions are relatively less common. The individual spinous processes and interspinous ligaments are palpated for tender-ness. Finally, the paravertebral muscles are palpated for areas of

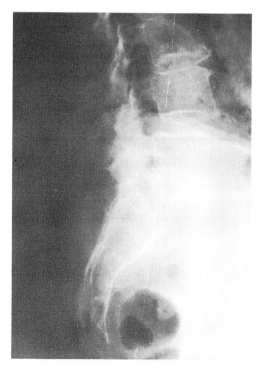

Figure 7a   Shelf in spondylolisthesis

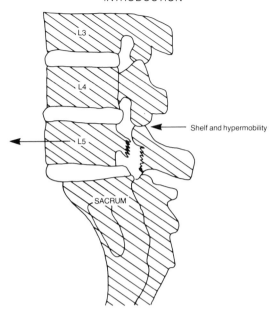

Figure 7b Diagram showing shelf and hypermobility at L_{4-5} in spondylolisthesis

tenderness and spasm. Absence of tenderness in a patient with definite back trouble suggests a lesion of one of the deeper structures, such as the disc; marked tenderness suggests either an apophyseal joint lesion or a ligamentous strain.

While the patient is in the prone position any marked wasting of the calves or thighs is noted, sacral and perianal sensation is tested and the ankle-jerks are best tested now. (This also gives a good opportunity to spot a sustained delayed relaxation, characteristic of hypothyroidism, see Chapter 8). The femoral nerve stretch test (FNS) is carried out by flexing the knee as far as it will go so that the heel approximates to the buttock and asking the patient to compare the discomfort produced at the front of the thigh with that on the opposite side (Figure 9). A more objective assessment of the FNS can be made by flexing the knee to a right angle and the examiner lifting the thigh off the table and noting at what angle pain and reflex muscle contraction impede the movement as compared with the good side (Figure 10).A positive FNS indicates a lesion of the upper lumbar roots (L_{1-4}).

This is a good opportunity to test the hip joints by another method. Rotation of the hips in the prone position is not usually affected in lumbar disorders, while in early osteoarthritis of the hip joints minor restriction of internal rotation and extension at the joints is often more readily demonstrated in the prone position.

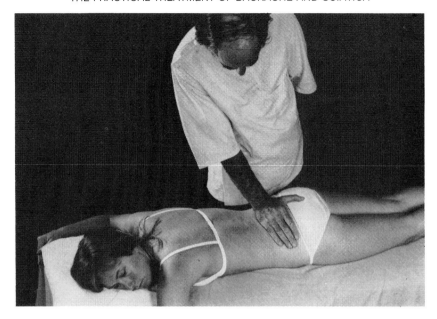

Figure 8   Springing the spine to detect muscle guarding

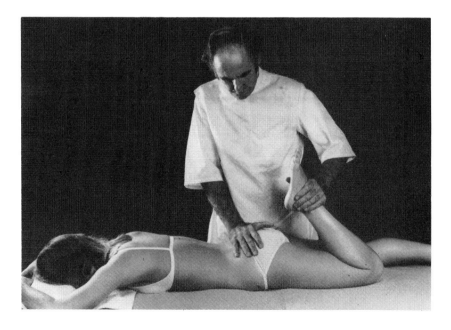

Figure 9   The femoral nerve stretch test by flexing the knee

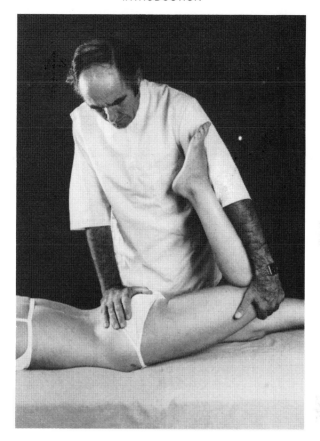

Figure 10   The femoral nerve stretch by extending the hip

Summary

Summarizing examination of the spine:

(a) EXAMINATION STANDING

Inspection:	Postural faults and deformities
	Differences in leg-lengths
	Knee and foot deformities
Lumbar spine movements:	Flexion, extension, side-flexion
	Blocking, painful arc
	Spinal hypermobility
	Plantar-flexion and dorsi-
	flexion of ankles

15

(b) EXAMINATION LYING SUPINE

Legs: Straight-leg-raising (SLR)
Knee-jerks
Quads and hamstrings
Ankle-jerks
Sensation
Plantar reflexes
Peripheral pulses

Sacro-iliac joints: Gapping, compression

Hip joints: Note fixed flexion deformity
Test movements

Abdomen: Note bladder, swellings etc.

(c) EXAMINATION SIDE-LYING

Spine rocking: Assessment of individual
movements of lumbar joints

(d) EXAMINATION LYING PRONE

Palpation of spine: Springing of vertebra and
sacrum
Palpate spinous processes and
ligaments
Palpate paravertebral muscles

Legs: Wasting of calves and thighs
Sacral and perianal sensation
Ankle-jerks
Femoral nerve stretch test
(FNS)
Hip joint rotation (check)

4. INVESTIGATING BACK PAIN

The great majority of backache sufferers, and particularly those with a first attack, do not need extensive investigation. Clinical examination will suffice to sort out the back pain syndrome and even an X-ray is not always mandatory. Indeed X-ray reports may be misleading – for example, 'lumbar spondylosis' is not necessarily the cause of the pain, as it is often symptomless; an associated intervertebral joint derangement may be the culprit, and this of course is not visible on the X-ray film.

It is generally accepted that *a young person with a first attack of backache need not necessarily have an X-ray or other investigations.* Obviously, investigations are required if symptoms persist in spite of treatment – for example, a young man may be developing sacro-iliitis, and sacro-iliac joint X-rays may therefore be revealing. In older patients it is important to exclude organic vertebral disease, such as bone tumours and metabolic bone disease, and in such cases at least a urine examination, X-rays of spine and pelvis, and blood-count and ESR are advisable. If ESR is raised the test should always be repeated; if it is still raised protein electrophoresis, immunoglobulins and acid and alkaline phosphates should be requested.

Radiology

Plain X-rays and radiculograms (myelograms) are the most commonly used radiological procedures. Bone scans and computed tomography are occasionally required.

Plain X-rays are usually taken in anteroposterior, lateral and coned lumbosacral views. They are not helpful in patients with recent disc lesions or intervertebral joint derangements, where they are often normal. With longstanding disc disease and degeneration there is reduction of the disc space and sometimes gas cavities are seen in the disc. X-rays are useful in diagnosing vertebral tumours, infections or ankylosing spondylitis, but do not always show these disorders, particularly in the early stages. Established osteoporosis or osteomalacia appears as loss of vertebral bone density with outstanding vertical trabeculae, but not until 30% of bone mass has been lost. Spondylosis, osteoarthritis, spondylolysis and spondylolisthesis are shown. In the latter condition oblique views may show breaks in the pars interarticularis (see Chapter 11.2).

Radiculograms (myelograms) (a) confirm and delineate disc prolapses, showing the extent of nerve root involvement and (b) illustrate space-occupying lesions in the spinal canal. In carrying out myelography the c.s.f. is routinely examined – a substantial increase in protein suggests a space-occuping lesion.

Bone scanning

The vertebrae, pelvis and sacro-iliac joints can be scanned to show the distribution and magnitude of the uptake of bone-seeking radioisotopes, particularly technetium 99m. The uptake depends on bone blood flow, bone metabolism and possibly osteoblastic activity (lesions of Paget's disease show up as 'hot spots'). Bone tumours, infections and sacro-iliitis can often be revealed by scanning when the plain X-ray is as yet normal. Vertebral fractures including osteoporotic crush fractures (but not osteoporosis without fracture) usually show moderately increased uptake, as does osteomalacia.

Computed axial tomography (CAT)

CAT scans may be useful in allowing cross-section visualization of the spine and soft tissues. Computed axial tomography is currently used for identifying spinal stenosis but the future may show a much wider field of usefulness in the context of elucidation of disc prolapses.

Blood investigations

Useful blood tests in back pain are: the erythocyte sedimentation rate (ESR), serum calcium and phosphorus, acid and alkaline phosphatases, protein electrophoresis, immunoglobulins and HLA antigens.

An ESR more than 25 mm/h (Westergren) in men or 30 mm/h in women may alert the physician to bone pathology, but it should be noted that rather higher ESRs are often encountered in 'normal' elderly patients.

A *high alkaline phosphatase* denotes bone formation following destruction, often as a result of tumour invasion. (Alternatively this may be found in liver disease when it is accompanied by elevation of other liver enzymes, especially Gamma G.T.)

A *high serum acid phosphatase* is usually (though not invariably) seen in prostatic carcinoma with bone secondaries. The formal-stable acid phosphatase (and not the formal labile phosphatase) is specific for prostatic disease.

The HLA-B27 histocompatability antigen is present in 95% patients with ankylosing spondylitis and a smaller though significant number of patients with other types of sero-negative spondarthritis (such as Reiter's disease or psoriatic arthritis with sacro-iliitis). Although HLA testing can be helpful in diagnosing pre-radiological sacro-iliitis (as might be suggested by spinal pain, morning stiffness and a very brisk response to anti-inflammatory drugs), this should not be a routine test in patients with backache, because HLA-B27 is present in 5–10% patients without sacro-iliitis or spondylitis, so a B27-positive patient without clinical or radiological evidence of sacro-iliitis is more likely *not* to have this condition at a given time.

Electromyography (e.m.g.)

It is important to know if more than one nerve root is involved when there is muscle weakness, as recovery often depends on this – single-root palsies usually recover fully, whereas double palsies often show delayed or incomplete recovery. Also, the finding of denervation potentials in the leg, buttock or paraspinal muscles can provide useful evidence for the extent of nerve root involvement by one or more prolapsed discs. Electromyography is also helpful in spinal stenosis where it often shows symmetrical multi-root denervation, more marked peripherally.

Vertebral biopsy

Open biopsy has been largely superseded by needle biopsy carried out under the image intensifier, using a needle incorporating a trephine so that a proper specimen is obtained. A high degree of diagnostic accuracy is obtained in this way, but the lesions are often patchy in distribution so that a mistaken negative biopsy may be obtained.

Summary of investigations

Note that *careful clinical examination* is essential in backache, and most patients do not need detailed laboratory investigation. Even a plain X-ray is not mandatory in a young adult having his first attack of backache.

(1) X-rays are useful in diagnosing spinal tumours and infections, ankylosing spondylitis, metabolic bone disease and vertebral instability such as spondylolisthesis. They do not show a recent disc lesion or other mechanical disorder of the spine.

(2) Radiculograms are used to confirm disc prolapses and space-occupying lesions of the spinal canal.

(3) Technetium bone scanning often may help to reveal tumour, infection, Paget's disease and sacro-iliitis before clear-cut radio-logical abnormalities appear.

(4) CAT scans are useful for identifying spinal stenosis, and may find a routine place in the investigation of prolapsed discs.

(5) A high ESR is a useful pointer to bone or joint disease in the spine.

(6) A high alkaline phosphatase denotes bone disease or liver disease. A high acid phosphatase occurs in prostatic cancer.

(7)   HLA-B27 occurs in 95% patients with ankylosing spondylitis, but it is found in 5–10% patients without sacro-iliitis so is not itself of diagnostic significance.

(8)   Electromyography helps in confirming the levels of lumbar nerve root involvement.

(9)   Vertebral biopsy may be helpful in confirming vertebral organic disease.

5.   PSYCHOLOGICAL FACTORS IN BACK PAIN

Patients with low back pain often have some psychological element to their symptoms. The personality, especially if prone to anxiety or depression, the domestic and work situation, and sometimes unwillingness to accept the ageing process – all colour the symptoms and the way in which the patient reacts to them. It is rare for backache to be *entirely* psychogenic, but equally it is exceptional for a person with unrelieved back trouble for many months to remain cheerful and well-adjusted. It follows that the physician often has an extremely difficult task in deciding exactly how much pain is organic and how much functional, yet it is vital to try to assess this on first seeing the patient. It is all too easy to label the patient that refuses to get better 'psychogenic', or to reinforce a patient's neurosis by continued complex investigations and treatment which may even culminate in a disastrous operation; the mildly neurotic patient can become a lifelong invalid after injudicious surgery.

There are four basic psychogenic factors which may so dominate a mild spinal lesion as to become the principal cause for the patient's continued illness. These are *anxiety, depression, secondary gain* (sometimes known as 'compensationitis'), and *malingering.*

Anxiety neurosis

In anxiety neurosis, backache is often accompanied by widespread pain in different parts of the body, in fact the patient will often come with a 'shopping list' of the symptoms 'to save your time, doctor'! Such patients embellish and dramatize their symptoms to illustrate that the pain is unbearable or excruciating, yet they have just walked normally into the consulting room. Sometimes paraesthesiae are described in non-anatomical distribution. These patients may have had a lot of previous treatment and say that each treatment has made them slightly worse. Examination may be difficult because of excessive and widespread tenderness leading to the patient wincing every time he or she is touched, or reluctance to make an effort to do the normal active movements required in the examination. Inconsistencies show up, such as that of the patient who cannot bend forward on standing but may be able to sit upright on a table and then bend forward while in that position at the doctor's request 'so that I can examine your back better'. Some of these patients respond well to anxiolytics such as small doses of diazepam (see Chapter 3.4).

Depression

The depressed patient may have some similarities to the above. In addition he will complain of excessive tiredness, and make statements such as 'I cannot stand my backache any longer unless you can do something, doctor'. Depressed patients are usually reluctant to go back to work and resume responsibility. A good result is often obtained from the use of antidepressive drugs such as amitriptyline (see Chapter 3.2).

Secondary gain

Secondary gain ('compensationitis') is becoming more frequent with increased litigation following accidents at work and on the road. Often the patient does not disclose that he has visited a solicitor, or is planning litigation, until he is presented with a diagnosis, so it is as well to be aware of possible litigation before discussing diagnosis and management. There are two useful clues to alert the physician to this situation: the first is that the patient, even though ambulatory, is often accompanied by a friend or spouse who insists on coming in to see the doctor as well. The second clue is that the patient often states the exact date of the injury in reply to the simple question: 'How long ago did this start?'

Almost without exception, treatment of chronic backache is unsatisfactory if a case of compensation is under way. Introspection over symptoms, bitterness towards the other side and the expectancy of damages exert so powerful an influence that these patients hang on to their pain until they have the money in the bank! The doctor's chief task is to urge a rapid settlement of the case once initial progress has come to a halt. The temptation to defer a further report to the solicitor and a final prognosis for another 6 months, in the hope that time will have resolved the symptoms, must be resisted. The longer the problem continues the more ingrained are the symptoms as the patient adapts his lifestyle to 'his bad back'. Courses of treatment that fail to help only serve to convince the patient that he has the symptoms for life and is entitled to big damages. It is better to supply a report and prognosis based on the physical signs rather than the symptoms, coupled with a frank statement to patients that experience shows that further treatment will be ineffective until litigation is out of the way. It is quite amazing how many lose interest in seeking further treatment once their case has been settled.

Malingering

Malingerers come in all shapes and sizes and their condition is often quite subconscious, malingering being a form of hysteria. A perfectly genuine back incident continues long after it should have resolved and is used to seek premature retirement, better housing or extra attention at home. The wife whose initial back trouble has resulted in her husband spending more time at home to do the housework, fetch the shopping and generally pay her more attention is reluctant to give up this satisfactory state of affairs! Men may find their 'chronic back' a useful face-saver to explain why they have failed to get on in life. Some may even choose to opt out of work if they have a boring job and prefer to pursue their hobbies (often more strenuous than their work) whilst relying on social security for income. For example, a 45-year-old man had been off work for 7 years when his elderly family physician retired and was replaced by a young and enthusiastic doctor who referred the patient because he felt that he was quite capable of following his employment as a clerk. The story was that he had an 'acute back' 7 years ago following lifting and had been placed in a plaster jacket for 3 months. On coming out of the plaster jacket he still found it painful to bend and his sympathetic doctor had continued issuing him off-work certificates until he became a 'chronic case'. He volunteered the information that he had managed very well on sickness benefit, his wife going out to work, until this young doctor came along! When asked what he did all day, his face lit up with enthusiasm as he described how he bred dogs and spent the morning exercising them, after which he found it necessary to lie down in the afternoon to help his back!

Summary of psychological factors in backache

Anxiety, depression or a combination of these are common in patients with backache and may greatly modify the symptoms, though purely 'psychogenic' backache is seen much less often.

The principle types of psychological reaction are anxiety, depression, secondary gain ('compensationitis') and malingering.

22

Anxiety and depression are sometimes effectively treated by appropriate drugs. This is not so in secondary gain and malingering, where the attitude of the physician to the patient is the all-important factor in management of these difficult situations.

References

Brady, L.P., Parker, L.B. and Waughan, J. (1969). An evaluation of the EMG in the diagnosis of the lumbar disc lesion. *J. Bone Joint Surg.*, **51**, 539

Finneson, B.E. (1980). *Low Back Pain.* (Philadelphia: J.B. Lippincott Co.)

Vernon–Roberts, B. (1980). Pathology and interrelation of intervertebral disc lesions, osteoarthrosis of apophyseal joints, lumbar spondylosis and low back pain. In Jayson, M. *The Lumbar Spine and Back Pain.* 2nd Edn. pp. 115-34 (London: Pitman Medical)

Williams, P.C. (1965) *The Lumbrosacral Spine.* (New York: McGraw Hill Book Co. Ltd)

2
Classification of Back Pain Syndromes

---

1. THE COMMON BACK PAIN SYNDROMES: APPROACH TO MANAGEMENT

Most backache and sciatica is basically due to progressive degeneration of the spinal joints, punctuated by acute episodes due to strain and other mechanical assaults. From this are derived a number of clearly defined syndromes and, although we may not understand the exact pathology in each case, these *common backache syndromes* form useful labels in discussing management:

Syndrome 1:   intervertebral joint derangement (IVJD)

Typically, after lifting – especially if there is a twisting element – the patient experiences sudden acute low back pain. There is no sciatica and straight-leg-raising is normal. Either forward- or backward-bending is usually blocked (but not both at once) and side-bending is usually more restricted on one side than the other. This type of syndrome is usually thought to be due to an internal derangement of an intervertebral (facet) joint (see Mooney and Robertson, 1976). The precipitating movement is often so trivial that it would be difficult to

24

believe that a muscle could have been torn; the degree of incapacity is far more than one would expect with a simple ligamentous strain - it seems to parallel the incapacity after a meniscus injury of the knee.

Although backache due to IVJD often clears up within a week, this is by no means invariable and quite a few patients are left with persistent mild pain after such an episode. This is the syndrome in which spinal manipulation is particularly effective and this should be the first treatment of choice. A rather poor second-best treatment is heat to relieve muscle spasm followed by exercises. One variety of acute lumbago to which one must be alert is where bilateral positive straight-leg-raising occurs in the absence of sciatica. Here there may be slight kyphosis, so that the patient is unable to stand up straight, and coughing aggravates the pain. This indicates a *central disc bulge* which often spontaneously goes on to a *lateral disc prolapse* with sciatica. Here the standard rotational manipulation may precipitate such a prolapse and is therefore contraindicated – the only safe manipulation in this condition is the 'vertical lift' which must be done in the sitting position if kyphosis is marked (see Chapter 5).

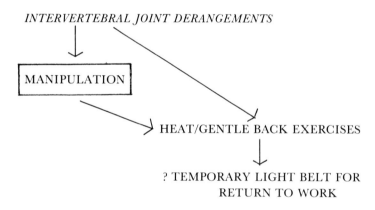

Diagram showing management of IVJ derangements

Syndrome 2: prolapsed intervertebral disc (PID)

In prolapsed intervertebral disc the pain may be initially in the leg (i.e. sciatica), but more often there is an initial episode of acute low back pain and after a few days sciatica develops together with relief of the low back pain. Sciatic pain is linear down the leg, quite sharp and is aggravated by coughing or sneezing. Frequently there are corresponding segmental paraesthesiae in the distribution of the nerve root or roots affected, this being less common in young people under 30. Motor involvement is often apparent in terms of muscle tone and slight wasting compared with the opposite side; frank muscle weakness is less common and often difficult to detect. There is diminution or loss of the knee-jerk in L_3 lesions, the ankle-jerk in S_1 lesions. Alteration in these reflexes is not apparent in 40% of patients, who have a 4th lumbar disc lesion involving the L_5 root, which is not associated with reflex changes. It is important to elicit signs of nerve root pressure as they leave no doubt about the diagnosis and level of the prolapse – limited straight-leg-raising by itself is not proof of disc prolapse (Table 2.1).

Patients with a prolapsed disc often have lumbar scoliosis due to muscle spasm, the so-called 'sciatic scoliosis'. Less frequently there is kyphosis on standing, with intense pain shooting down the leg on backward bending. If a patient is unable to extend the spine to reach the vertical position the prognosis for recovery with conservative treatment is poor, as this indicates a large protrusion and it is more likely that surgical treatment will be needed.

The acute disc should always be initially treated with a few days' complete bedrest. If sciatica persists the choice can then be made of either a caudal epidural injection (see Chapter 6) or a course of inter-mittent lumbar traction in the physiotherapy department (see Chapter 4). Failure to respond to these will indicate the need for admission to hospital for complete bed rest and continuous pelvic traction (see Chapter 10). A small number of cases does not respond to conservative treatment in hospital and will require surgery (Chapter 11), but occasionally manipulation under anaesthetic helps this group (Chapter 5).

Beware the patient with sciatica and difficulty passing water. This is usually a manifestation of (a) loss of the normal bladder sensation and (b) weakness of the bladder wall giving loss of power to mictur-ate. This may also apply to defecation and in such cases there is often

Table 2.1 Chart of nerve root levels: clincial features

Nerve root	Pain	Numbness	Principal muscle weakness	Reflex
L_3	Anterior thigh	Anterior thigh and medial aspect knee	Quadriceps	Knee ↓
L_4	Anterior thigh and shin	Anterior shin	Quadriceps	Knee ↓
L_5	Lateral calf and dorsum of foot	Big toe	Extensor hallucis longus	Normal
S_1	Back of calf	Outer side of foot	Plantar flexors	Ankle ↓

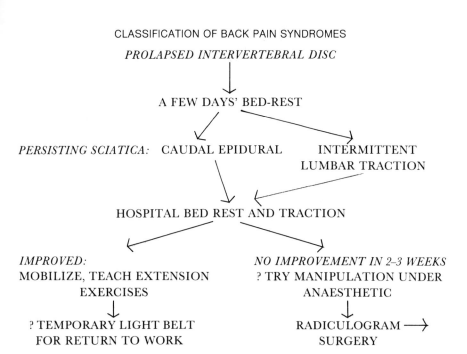

PROLAPSED INTERVERTEBRAL DISC

A FEW DAYS' BED-REST

PERSISTING SCIATICA: CAUDAL EPIDURAL INTERMITTENT LUMBAR TRACTION

HOSPITAL BED REST AND TRACTION

IMPROVED:
MOBILIZE, TEACH EXTENSION
EXERCISES

? TEMPORARY LIGHT BELT
FOR RETURN TO WORK

NO IMPROVEMENT IN 2–3 WEEKS
? TRY MANIPULATION UNDER
ANAESTHETIC

RADICULOGRAM ⟶
SURGERY

Diagram showing basic management of lumbar disc lesions

loss of pain sensation over the perineum – known as 'saddle anaesthesia'. These are the symptoms of the *cauda equina syndrome*, where there is compression of the S_2 nerve root by a prolapsed L_5 disc, usually a large midline central protrusion which causes bilateral sciatica owing to pressure on the S_1 roots as well. There may be marked weakness of one or more muscle groups, often bilaterally. In the cauda equina syndrome no time must be lost in facilitating immediate surgical decompression of the involved nerve roots if function is to be restored.

Syndrome 3: chronic spinal osteoarthritis

Backache and sciatica are usually due to progressive degeneration of spinal joints punctuated by acute episodes as already described. Fortunately, the majority of patients recover from acute episodes and are comparatively free of symptoms for long periods. However, occasionally after one or two acute episodes the patient is left with continuous low back pain, sciatica, or both. A typical story is that since the last acute episode the patient is left with moderate low back pain which allows him to get about but makes it difficult for him to do bending jobs, to stand for long periods and to sit in a low chair such as

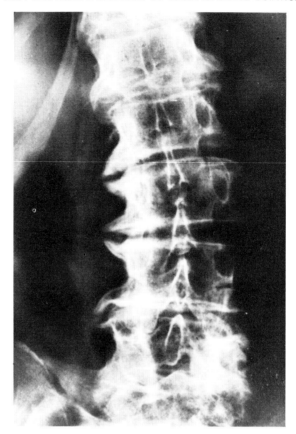

Figure 11 Anterior spondylosis, showing horizontal osteolytes (lipping) and narrow inter-vertebral discs

the car seat. This is chronic spinal osteoarthritis, which develops as follows: owing to loss of disc material the annulus becomes lax, giving rise to instability and hence pain from ligaments and the capsules of facet-joints. The formation of osteophytic spurs leads to narrowing of the spinal canal and the lateral nerve root recesses and may be responsible for nerve root irritation or pressure. In overweight lordotic patients (especially if there is a family history of osteo-arthritis) the posterior facet joints become osteoarthritic, with bony overgrowths helping to reduce the size of the lateral recesses of the spinal canal.

Chronic spinal osteoarthritis is of two varieties, and the two may coexist. The first is *anterior spondylosis*, the wear-and-tear process involving the anterior vertebrae and the discs: osteophytes are seen in the X-ray (Figure 11), the discs are narrow and may contain air. This type of spondylosis is often amenable to treatment by physiotherapy and manipulation. The second type of osteoarthritis is *posterior (facet) joint osteoarthritis,* a true synovial joint osteoarthritis which is much more difficult to treat effectively by conventional means, such measures as facet injections and radiofrequency lesions (see Chapter 7.6) sometimes being required for relief of pain.

In considering the management of spinal osteoarthritis, the duration of continuous back pain is important. If this is less than a year, especially if the patient is under 60, energetic conservative treatment should be tried to restore the spine to its state before the last acute episode. If the spinal movements are generally restricted, manipulation and exercise may restore some movement. If morning stiffness is a marked feature, one of the anti-inflammatory drugs may help. If the main complaint is leg pain (sciatica or referred pain to the legs) and there is a good range of lumbar movements without muscle spasm, the patient often benefits from a course of intermittent lumbar traction as an outpatient. However, where symptoms have remained unchanged for more than a year the chances of improvement with such conservative treatment diminish considerably. Disc surgery is not normally considered in these cases – usually only the sciatica is relieved, the low back pain component remaining unchanged. If the main problem is backache and back movements are poor, one aims at trying to relieve this by provision of a well-fitting lumbar corset and prescription of suitable analgesics.

Be on the watch for two groups of patients in this category who can easily be labelled 'functional'. The first is the young person in the 25–35 years age group who complains of gradually increasing backache, usually in the upper lumbar spine. Look for reversal of the normal lumbar lordosis in the upper lumbar area and marked stiffness of this region on springing the spine in the prone position. X-rays often suggest that these patients have adolescent osteochondritis (Scheuermann's disease) leading to wedging of the upper lumbar vertebrae and scattered Schmorl's nodes. The onset of degenerative changes with disc narrowing and osteophytic lipping is undoubtedly accelerated in these patients and, being young, they demand quite a bit from their backs and so frequently develop pain in these degenerative joints.

The second group, less common but nevertheless important, comprises patients who complain of numbness and weakness of one or both legs together with mild pain on walking any distance. These are usually in the age group 45–60 years and are describing a form of *neurogenic claudication,* where a nerve root or the cauda equina is compressed by a disc or spondylotic process. Some of these patients have spinal stenosis and may require surgery, though lumbar traction can be helpful in many cases (see Chapter 11).

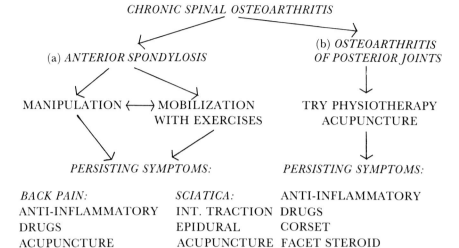

CHRONIC SPINAL OSTEOARTHRITIS

(a) *ANTERIOR SPONDYLOSIS*

(b) *OSTEOARTHRITIS OF POSTERIOR JOINTS*

MANIPULATION ⟷ MOBILIZATION WITH EXERCISES

TRY PHYSIOTHERAPY ACUPUNCTURE

PERSISTING SYMPTOMS:

PERSISTING SYMPTOMS:

BACK PAIN:
ANTI-INFLAMMATORY
DRUGS
ACUPUNCTURE
CORSET (IF SYMPTOMS
> 1 YEAR)

SCIATICA:
INT. TRACTION
EPIDURAL
ACUPUNCTURE

ANTI-INFLAMMATORY
DRUGS
CORSET
FACET STEROID
INJECTIONS
RADIOFREQUENCY LESIONS

Diagram showing basic management of chronic spinal osteoarthritis

Syndrome 4:   ligamentous (postural) backache

This is pure, chronic backache, there being no history of acute episodes but gradual onset of a dull ache in the back rather than sharp pains (Howes and Isdale, 1971). At first the pain comes on only when in a set posture, such as standing or sitting still for long periods, and in contrast the patient may be able to dash around and even play tennis or similar games without trouble. The pain first comes on in the latter half of the day, and as the condition develops it starts earlier in the day until eventually there is a continuous backache, rather similar to the aching produced by flat feet. Patients with ligamentous backache usually have poor posture with a reversed lumbar curve ('sway back') and poor muscle tone. There may be a precipitating factor, such as recent pregnancy which involves a combination of stretched spinal ligaments, tiredness and an increasingly heavy infant to pick up, or else there is a recent illness necessitating several weeks in bed and hence loss of muscle tone, or a new job involving standing all day.

It seems likely that ligamentous backache denotes breakdown in the normal ligamentous–muscular relationship, so that the postural tensions fall on the ligaments as they cannot be served by normal muscle tone. Examination shows no evidence of articular derangement, there being a good range of lumbar movements (which indeed may be excessive in the hypermobility or 'loose back' syndrome (Figure

12) and, other than hypermobility, the only positive sign is tenderness on palpating the interspinous and sacro-iliac ligaments. Management consists of supplying a temporary lumbar corset, (which is comparable to giving arch supports for flat feet), together with a regime of gentle back exercises to improve muscle tone including regular walking or swimming. (Intensive back exercises only aggravate ligamentous pain.) Advice on posture includes ensuring that the lumbar spine is supported and not allowed to sag when sitting and avoiding the half-bending position which puts extra stretch on the lumbar ligaments. Some patients are helped by acupuncture (see Chapter 7) and if these measures fail to relieve pain, sclerosing injections to the interspinous ligaments can be considered (see Chapter 6).

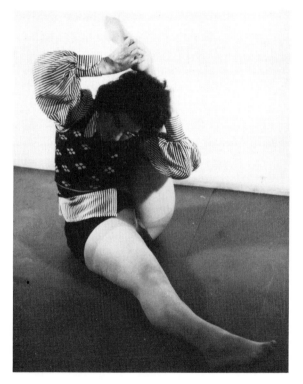

Figure 12 Demonstration of excessively mobile joints in the hypermobility syndrome

Summary

The common back pain syndromes are as follows.

(1) *Intervertebral joint derangements.* Sudden pain, no sciatica. Straight-leg-raising (SLR) normal. Blocking of spinal movement. Spinal manipulation effective. (If bilateral SLR reduced or positive:

LIGAMENTOUS (POSTURAL) BACKACHE

↓

TEMPORARY SMALL CORSET + TEACH BACK EXERCISES
+ CORRECT POSTURE

↓

? ACUPUNCTURE

↓

? SCLEROSING INJECTIONS

Diagram showing management of ligamentous backache

beware central disc prolapse, manipulation contraindicated.

(2) *Prolapsed intervertebral disc.* Sciatica, or back pain progressing to sciatica, segmental paraesthesiae, sometimes weakness. Reflex changes (except in L_4 lesions). Beware cauda equina compression – dysuria, saddle anaesthesia, bilateral sciatica and weakness.

(3) *Chronic spinal osteoarthritis.* Low back pain, sometimes sciatica or referred pain, no paraesthesiae. (a) Anterior spondylosis (easily treated), (b) posterior (facet) spondylosis (treated with difficulty). Improve spinal movements if symptoms of short duration, traction helps sciatica when movements are good. Corset if symptoms of long duration and back movements are poor. Young persons with increasing upper lumbar backache may have osteochondritis (Scheuermann's disease). Patients with neurogenic claudication have cauda equina or root cord compression by disc, spondylosis or spinal stenosis.

(4) *Ligamentous (postural) backache.* Chronic backache on standing or sitting, poor posture, poor muscle tone. Normal back movements (excessive in hypermobility syndrome). Treated with temporary corset, back exercises and postural advice. Acupuncture may help. Sclerosing injections occasionally required.

2. LESS COMMON CAUSES OF BACK PAIN

Although the vast majority of patients with backache have a mechanical cause for their symptoms and belong to one of the common syndromes as above, one must always be on the alert for the occasional case due to a pathological disorder such as a vertebral tumour, Paget's disease of bone or ankylosing spondylitis. Important examples include the elderly patient with a history of malignancy and a first attack of back pain – which is unrelenting and severe at night, accompanied by loss of weight and malaise. When it comes to examination of the spine the physician will be alerted by the odd sign which does not 'fit in' with the usual picture of disc disease or osteoarthritis or else an elderly woman has an osteoporotic compression fracture of a vertebra which has followed minor trauma, such as opening a sash window, and may mimic an intervertebral joint derangement. Such patients may have good spinal movements on examination, but they climb onto the examination couch with difficulty because this involves a levering effect on the fractured vertebra; they often emit a series of grunts while attempting this and, once lying prone on the couch, springing of the vertebrae shows obvious muscle guarding at the level of the lesion!

Classification

The less common causes of back pain can be classified as follows:

(1) *Traumatic conditions* (other than disc lesions/joint derangements)
  Vertebral fractures (of either normal or pathological bone)

(2) *Congenital defects*
  Congenital scoliosis
  Spina bifida
  Spondylolysis
  Spondylolisthesis
  Spinal stenosis

(3) *Acquired deformities*
  Kyphosis (e.g. following spinal osteochondritis, tuberculosis)
  Scoliosis (e.g. following poliomyelitis)

(4) *Infectious lesions*, e.g.
  Tuberculosis
  Osteomyelitis
  Brucellosis

(5) *Arthritis* (other than osteoarthritis/spondylosis)
  Ankylosing spondylitis and other types of sero-negative spondarthritis
  Rheumatoid arthritis (rare in spine other than cervical region)

(6) *Spinal osteochondritis* (Scheuermann's disease)

(7) *Neoplasms*, e.g.
  Benign tumours (osteoma, angioma)
  Malignant tumours (rarely primary bone tumours, usually secondary)

Myeloma, Hodgkin's disease and leukaemic infiltration

(8) *Metabolic bone disease,* principally
     Osteoporosis
     Osteomalacia
     Hyperparathyroidism

(9) *Paget's disease of bone*

(10) *Space-occupying lesions of spinal canal*
     Principally tumours or inflammatory lesions of bone, meninges
     or spinal cord

In practice, the commonest pathological disorders are *ankylosing spondylitis* in the young, *secondary vertebral tumours* in the middle-aged and elderly and *osteoporosis* in the over-60s.

Back pain referred from visceral disorders

It is very unusual, if not rare, for back pain to be derived from visceral disease. Some examples are renal disease (e.g. pyelonephritis), uterine or ovarian disease, pancreatic disease (pancreatitis or carcinoma), chronic duodenal ulceration penetrating the pancreas and a large aneurysm of the descending aorta which abuts against the vertebral bodies. It is now generally accepted that gynaecological conditions such as retroversion and prolapse are rarely, if ever, responsible for backache. However, heavy and prolonged menstrual periods may aggravate mild chronic backache, and treatment of the pelvic disorder (such as hysterectomy) may lead to alleviation of backache.

Investigation of organic back pain

The principal investigations required in patients with back pain considered to be due to one of the above conditions are:

(1) Plain X-rays of spine and pelvis

(2) Special radiography (tomography, radiculogram, scanning)

(3) Blood-count and ESR

(4) Serum calcium, phosphorus, alkaline (and in males acid) phosphatase

(5) Serum proteins and electrophoresis

(6) Immunoglobulins

(7) Tests for bacterial antibodies (e.g. ASO, anti-staphyloccocal antibodies, brucella antibodies)

(8) HLA antigens (HLA-B27 in ankylosing spondylitis and sero-negative spondarthropathies (see Chapter 1)

(9) Vertebral biopsy, to confirm bone tumour or infection. Biopsy of an iliac crest is useful to confirm myelomatosis or osteomalacia

(10) Bone marrow biopsy (in myeloma and reticuloses)

Management of patients with organic vertebral disease

Spinal tuberculosis

The X-ray shows destructive changes of discs as well as adjoining vertebrae, and paravertebral cold abscesses may be seen (Figure 13), Essential treatment is prolonged rest and antituberculous drugs.

Osteomyelitiis

Staphycoccal infection is not uncommon. Often X-rays are normal for the first few months, the ESR is high and there is a rising titre of anti-staphylococcal antibodies. Muscle spasm adjacent to the lesion is marked and the temperature may be raised. Blood culture may be

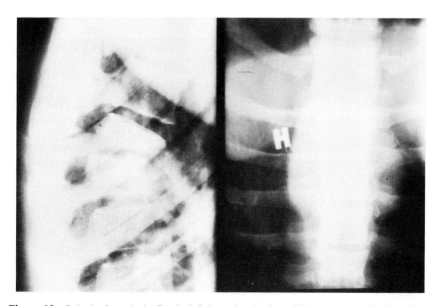

Figure 13 Spinal tuberculosis. On the left (anterior view) a cold abscess extending laterally is seen. The right view shows wedge-shaped destruction of a vertebra with adjacent disc destruction

positive, open or closed vertebral biopsy may be required. Treatment is by immobilization and long-term antibiotics.

Ankylosing spondylitis

This should be suspected particularly in young men presenting with back pain and morning stiffness, but it can be picked up in older patients and it is not uncommon in women where it is often of a mild nature. Some patients have iritis or a history of inflammatory eye disease. Initially the sacro-iliac and spinal X-rays may be normal, and the diagnosis suspected (though not proven) by the clinical features along with a high ESR and the presence of HLA-B27. Early sacro-iliac changes (such as irregularity, widening, narrowing or para-articular sclerosis) may be seen in later films (Figure 14). Bony ankylosis with complete loss of definition of the sacro-iliac joints (Figure 15) is a late change, as is ligamentous calcification and the classical X-ray appearance of the 'bamboo spine'.

The basic treatment of ankylosing spondylitis entails:

(1) Non-steroidal anti-inflammatory agents (more effective than simple analgesics) to relieve pain and stiffness. Phenylbutazone is probably the most potent drug in spondylitis and may be given

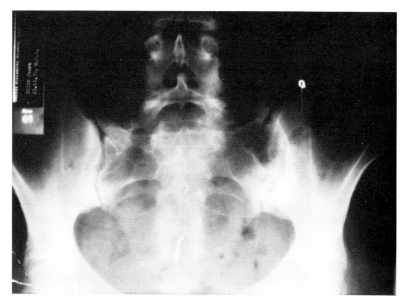

Figure 14 Early unilateral sacro-iliitis, showing irregular narrowing of sacro-iliac joint and para-articular sclerosis

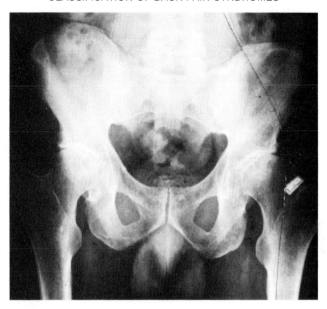

Figure 15 Advanced ankylosing spondylitis, showing fusion of sacro-iliac joints (note also hip-joint involvement)

intermittently in small doses, but if prolonged therapy is required it is safer to switch to another anti-inflammatory drug such as naproxen, indomethacin, flurbiprofen or piroxicam.

(2) Spinal exercises to retain mobility and prevent deformity. Patients are taught to carry out a full regime of exercises for the whole spine, also breathing exercises, at least once daily. Hydrotherapy and swimming are helpful to mobilize the spine, especially in patients immobilized in bed for even short periods as they stiffen up easily.

(3) General education. It is important for the patient to understand the nature of the disease and the need for drugs and regular exercise. Owing to the hereditary nature of ankylosing spondylitis genetic counselling may be advisable.

(4) Intra-articular steroid injections are useful for involved peripheral joints (e.g. knees), associated soft-tissue lesions (e.g. plantar fasciitis) and may be effective when given into a persistently-active sacro-iliac joint. (Systemic steroids are very rarely required. They are occasionally useful as a temporary measure to tide the patient over a very acute exacerbation, but

should never be continued indefinitely as they are conducive to osteoporosis and eventually vertebral fractures.)

(5) Radiotherapy. While the pain of ankylosing spondylitis often responds well to deep X-ray therapy, this is rarely given because of the predisposition to leukaemia in patients so treated.

(6) Surgery. Hip replacement gives excellent results in patients with progressive ankylosis of one or both hip joints. Very occasionally spinal osteotomy is carried out when there is severe flexion deformity of the spine resulting from longstanding, poorly treated spondylitis.

Osteochondritis (Scheurmann's disease)

This is probably the commonest cause of back pain in adolescents, and involves mainly the lower thoracic/upper lumbar spine. It is a

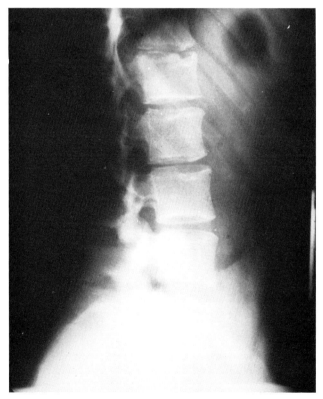

Figure 16 Spinal osteochondritis, showing Schmorl's node in antero-superior aspect of body of of L2.

non-specific inflammatory condition in which Schmorl's nodes are seen in the X-ray (Figure 16) and which is usually self-limiting, but severe cases should have prolonged complete bed rest as there may be extension through the epiphyseal plates causing erosion of the antero-superior and antero-inferior aspects of the vertebral bodies leading to wedging and consequent kyphosis. Patients with osteochondritis seem to be unduly prone to develop spondylosis in the affected areas later on, and many young adults with backache may have had mild osteochondritis in their teens.

Secondary vertebral neoplasms

There is evidence that the formation of prostaglandin E_2 by bone tumours causes both resorption and pain. It is therefore always worthwhile trying prostaglandin-inhibiting anti-inflammatory drugs, such as indomethacin. A concerted attempt should always be made to find the primary tumour – most often in the lungs, breast, kidney, prostate or thyroid. Prostatic secondaries are sclerotic rather than bone-destroying. The acid phosphatase is raised, but not invariably so, and a large, hard prostate palpated *per rectum* is the best indicator of neoplasm. The diagnosis can be confirmed by prostate biopsy and treatment with oestrogens (e.g. stilboestrol, up to 3 mg daily) is often rewarding, but relapse usually occurs within a few years. Myeloma is usually revealed by electrophoresis or immunoelectrophoresis (showing an abnormal paraprotein) or by sternal/iliac crest biopsy; initial X-rays may be negative, as back pain can precede radiological changes by many months. The short-term prognosis of myeloma treated with immunosuppressive agents (e.g. melphalan together with systemic steroids) is often good.

Metabolic bone disease

The most important type of osteoporosis is *postmenopausal osteoporosis* (with eventual compression fractures of the vertebrae (Figure 17). It is fashionable to treat this with oestrogens, keeping a watch for withdrawal bleeding, or else calcium preparations are advised. A typical regime is Sandocal (calcium gluconate with sodium and potassium bicarbonate) 3 tablets daily, ethinyloestradiol 20 μg daily for 21 days and norethisterone 350 μg for 7 days of the cycle. *Osteomalacia* usually results from vitamin D deficiency, often dietary or due to malabsorption, which can be corrected with small doses of vitamin D (2000–4000 units daily) or 1α-hydroxycholecalciferol. Osteomalacia also may occur in malabsorption states and in chronic renal or liver disease (Figure 18). *Primary hyperparathyroidism,* due to parathyroid adenoma,

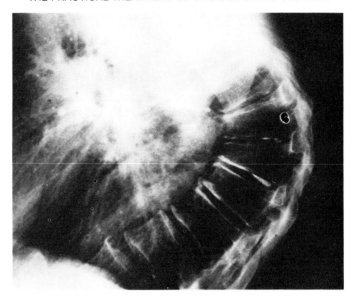

Figure 17 Wedge-shaped vertebrae due to compression fractures in osteoporosis. Note calcification in intervertebral discs – an additional source of back pain

may cause generalized osteoporosis or cystic changes in the vertebrae; active cases may require parathyroidectomy.

Paget's disease of the spine

This disorder is characterized by concurrent bone absorption and new bone formation. Vertebral lesions should not necessarily be deemed to be the cause of back pain as they are often symptomless and picked up in routine X-rays of the spine and pelvis. Active Paget's disease (as shown by high serum alkaline phosphatase) is associated with bone pain, occasionally acute due to associated stress fractures. Lesions may encroach on the intervertebral discs and are therefore a rare cause of sciatica due to nerve root involvement. Vertebral X-rays show patchy increase of bone density with expansion of the cortex. Treatment using calcitonin, editronate (a diphosphonate) or a combination of these drugs often gives satisfactory relief of pain and a corresponding drop in the serum alkaline phosphatase.

Summary: less common causes of back pain

(1) It is again emphasized that back pain is usually due to intervertebral joint derangements, disc lesions or osteoarthritis.

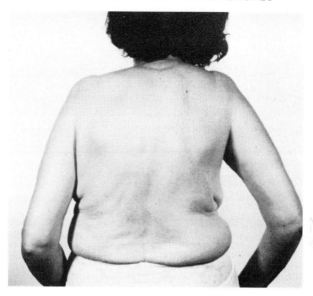

Figure 18 Kyphoscoliosis giving shortened stature in a patient with osteomalacia

Much less commonly it is due to vertebral fractures, congenital defects such as scoliosis, acquired spinal deformities, vertebral infections, ankylosing spondylitis or sacro-iliitis, vertebral osteochondritis, neoplasms, myelomatosis, osteoporosis or osteomalacia, Paget's disease of bone or space-occupying lesions of the spinal canal. It is most unusual for disorders of the viscera to be the primary cause of back pain.

(2) Useful investigations in back pain suspected to be due to organic disease are radiography, scanning, ESR, immunoelectrophoresis, HLA typing, serum calcium, phosphorus and acid/alkaline phosphatases. Myelography, bone-marrow and vertebral biopsy are occasionally indicated.

(3) Ankylosing spondylitis usually presents in young men with back pain and stiffness. Treatment includes non-steroidal anti-inflammatory drugs, exercise therapy, steroid injections to active peripheral joints and surgery for hip ankylosis.

(4) Osteochondritis, a cause of back pain in teenagers and patients in their twenties, is usually self-limiting, but occasionally it is progressive leading to spinal deformity.

(5) Vertebral neoplasms are nearly always secondary, coming from the chest, breast, kidney, prostate or thyroid. Hormone-

dependent tumours such as prostatic carcinoma can often be controlled by oestrogens, others (including myeloma) by chemotherapy.

(6) Postmenopausal osteoporosis is best treated with oestrogens. Osteomalacia is treated with vitamin D or one of its analogues.

(7) Paget's disease of the vertebrae or pelvis may cause bone pain. Calcitonin or editronate therapy is often effective.

References

Howes, R.J. and Isdale, I.C. (1971). The loose back – an unrecognised syndrome. *Rheum. Phys. Med.*, **11**, 72

Moll, J.M.H. (1980). *Ankylosing Spondylitis*. (Edinburgh and London: Churchill Livingstone)

Mooney, V. and Robertson, J. (1976). The facet syndrome. *Clin. Orthop.*, **115**, 146

3
Drugs in the Treatment of Back Pain

Drugs and medicines are not a mainline treatment of backache and sciatica, but they form an important adjunct to treatment in two respects. Firstly, they provide immediate pain relief while more specific treatment is awaited. Secondly, drugs help to facilitate such measures as physiotherapy and manipulation – by relieving pain, relaxing muscles, allaying anxiety and thereby increasing confidence.

Drugs used in backache and sciatica are:

(1) *Analgesics*. These may be classified as:
    (a) Mild analgesics (e.g. paracetamol)
    (b) Moderately powerful analgesics (e.g. dihydrocodeine)
    (c) Very powerful analgesics (e.g pethidine)

(2) *Sedatives, hypnotics and muscle relaxants*

(3) *Psychotropic drugs*. These are principally:
    (a) Anxiolytic drugs
    (b) Antidepressive drugs

(4) *Anti-inflammatory drugs* – principally non-steroidal anti-inflammatory drugs (abbreviated as NSAID)

1. ANALGESICS

The physician's first aim is to relieve pain and to this end he must think of a suitable analgesic. He will decide whether a mild, moderately powerful or very strong analgesic drug is required. Aspirin and paracetamol are examples of mild analgesics – up to 12 aspirins (3.6 g) or eight paracetamols (4 g) a day may be given. Aspirin and paracetamol are conveniently combined with each other as benorylate (Benoral) 10 ml twice-daily, which enables a high dose of aspirin to be accepted by most patients. Diflunisal (Dolobid) is another mild anal-

43

gesic which can be given in b.d. dosage (250–500 b.d.). Should a rather more powerful analgesic be required one can consider codeine phosphate or Panadeine Co. (paracetamol 500 mg with codeine phosphate 8 mg in each tablet). Contrary to what is sometimes thought, dextropropoxyphene (in Distalgesic or Cosalgesic) is only a mild-to-moderate analgesic, well accepted by some but not all patients. It must be remembered that dependency may occur with this drug and there are occasionally withdrawal symptoms. It can be dangerous when taken with alcohol.

In considering analgesics for more severe cases of back pain, and particularly for severe sciatica, it is often necessary to think of powerful analgesics such as dihydrocodeine, pentazocine, buprenorphine or even dipipanone. These should always be prescribed on a p.r.n. (as required) basis and not taken regularly throughout the day. Dihydrocodeine (DF 118) is useful – one or two 30 mg tablets should be taken 4- or 6-hourly as required. Unfortunately this drug is not tolerated well in all patients and tends to constipate, an undesirable effect when bowel action is already a problem in patients with acute disc lesions. Pentazocine (Fortral) 25–50 mg t.i.d. p.r.n. is rather less powerful and causes unacceptable dizziness in ambulant patients. Buprenorphine (Temgesic) is taken sublingually (one 0.2 mg tablet p.r.n.) – it is powerful, often well accepted and non-addictive. Dipipanone (in Diconal, which also contains the antiemetic cyclizine) should be used only in cases of intractable back pain. It should be prescribed cautiously as there is a risk of addiction, and should never be given to elderly patients or those with a history of or incipient cardiovascular disease as it is a respiratory depressant. In such cases in general practice pethidine is probably to be preferred (though this is not often used in hospital-treated cases). Except for patients suffering from back pain associated with malignancy, drugs such as morphine and diamorphine (heroin) should be avoided for obvious reasons.

2. SEDATIVES, HYPNOTICS AND MUSCLE RELAXANTS

Night sedatives are important in the management of patients with disc lesions and severe back pain in general. The best sedative may well be a single dose of a tranquillizer, such as nitrazepam (Mogadon), diazepam (Valium) or chlorazepate (Tranxene). More distinct sedation is given by temazepam (Normison), or – rather longer-acting, so there is more likely to be a 'hangover' effect next morning – flurazepam (Dalmane). An antihistamine such as promethazine (Phenergan) is often used for its sedative effect in children. Barbiturates (taken regularly by millions in a bygone era), should be avoided owing to their strongly-addictive effects, but it is inadvisable to try to wean patients accustomed to taking a barbiturate off their tablets as the whole situation could be greatly aggravated by withdrawal problems.

In the treatment of the acute disc or other severe back pain it can be very helpful to prescribe a so-called muscle relaxant drug together with analgesics. These usually have a central action which reduces muscle tone, but one cannot rule out the possibility that tranquillization, such as is provided by diazepam (Valium), chlormezanone (as in Lobak) or meprobamate (as in Equagesic), is also a factor.

3. PSYCHOTROPIC DRUGS

These are mainly anxiolytic and antidepressive drugs. It is very important to assess the degree of anxiety and depression in every case of back pain (as pointed out in Chapter 1.5) and to actively treat cases where these factors are relevant.

Anxiolytic drugs should be considered in all patients with backache even if they are not very obviously tense and anxious, because of their role in doubling as muscle relaxants. It is absolutely essential that a patient with a disc lesion who is lying flat on his back for days at a time, whether or not he is on continuous traction, must be pushed to full mental relaxation. Relaxant drugs can also be helpful for patients having outpatient physiotherapy if prescribed an hour before treatment commences. Pain which does not respond adequately to analgesics may be relieved by adding a small regular dose of an anxiolytic, such as diazepam. This, the most commonly-used, long-acting benzodiazepine anxiolytic, should be given for limited periods only, owing to the development of tolerance. Also, it would seem that the drug has a particularly depressing effect when given over a long period – indeed, it is sometimes wrongly prescribed in depressive states – it is certainly not an antidepressant. Other anxiolytics include chlordiazepoxide (Librium), chlorazepate (Tranxene), lorazepam (Ativan) and oxazepam (Serenid) – the last two are shorter-acting.

It is rarely necessary to prescribe the so-called 'major tranquillizers' for patients with low back pain. These include chlorpromazine (Largactil), trifluoperazine (Stelazine), thioridazine (Melloril) and flupenthixol (Fluanxol). Should these be indicated, small doses should be prescribed for only very short periods.

Unlike anxiolytics, which are given almost routinely for backache, *antidepressant drugs* are only indicated for patients who are definitely depressed, not only by extrinsic factors but also perhaps by the continued presence of the backache itself. With these drugs fashions change, and there is no hard-and-fast rule about which are the best at any given point in time. Rheumatologists usually prefer tricyclic drugs (such as amitriptyline) to monoamine-oxidase inhibitors (MAOI) for routine use, though psychiatrists may disagree. A good method of prescribing amitriptyline is to give 50 mg at night, then build up the dose if necessary. However, the drug should be introduced in small doses of 10–25 mg in elderly patients. This has sedative properties, and is more useful in agitated than in retarded depression, where imipramine 25 mg t.i.d. may be preferred to amitriptyline as it is less sedative. All these drugs have a latent period of 1–3 weeks before their antidepressive effect is observed, though the sedative effect of amitriptyline is usually immediate. The elderly sometimes tolerate mianserin (Bolvidon) better than amitriptyline as they are often prone to the hypotensive effect of tricyclics. In these patients an additional antidepressive effect may be provided by adding tryptophan, such as in Optimax (= tryptophan 550 mg with pyridoxine and ascorbic acid).

4. ANTI-INFLAMMATORY DRUGS

Except for purely *inflammatory* types of backache (notably ankylosing spondylitis and other types of sero-negative spondarthritis) where they are extremely effective, it is not clear whether or not non-steroidal anti-inflammatory drugs (NSAID) have a very useful part to play in the common types of backache. Certainly they are effective for episodes of *acute osteoarthritis* of the apophyseal joints, which respond to short (3–10 day) courses of a non-steroidal anti-inflammatory drug such as indomethacin or naproxen. These drugs only occasionally are helpful for patients with *chronic backache*, where an initially moderate dose should be reduced to the lowest possible maintenance dose, e.g. indomethacin 25 mg every night. Stiffness is also relieved, this being especially common in patients over 45 years of age. However, some caution should be exercised, as it has been suggested that indomethacin and probably others can be deleterious as they inhibit bone and cartilage metabolism and particularly inhibit proteoglycan synthesis in disc tissue. Certainly NSAIDs have no proven beneficial effect in patients with *acute disc lesions*.

Non-steroidal anti-inflammatory drugs are principally carboxylic acids or enolic acids. These are classified as follows, well-known examples being given in brackets:

Carboxylic acids:
    (a) Salicylic acids (aspirin and derivatives)
    (b) Phenylacetic acids (diclofenac, fenclofenac)

(c) Indole acetic acids (indomethacin)

(d) Propionic acids (ibuprofen, naproxen, flurbiprofen, fenprofen, ketoprofen)

(e) Fenamic acids (flufenamic and mefenamic acids)

Enolic acids:

(f) Pyrazolones (phenylbutazone, azapropazone)

(g) Oxicams (piroxicam)

One example in each group will be briefly described.

(a) Aspirin. This is anti-inflammatory in full dosage, but is used mainly for its analgesic effect in patients with backache (see Section 1, Analgesics).

(b) Diclofenac (Voltarol) 25 mg t.i.d. This, an NSAID of proven efficacy, has the advantage of not being protein-binding, so (unlike most others) it does not interfere with the action of anti-coagulant drugs.

(c) Indomethacin. This is the best-tried and probably the most powerful NSAID. However, side-effects (principally cerebral) are common, especially in the elderly. It is advisable to start with 50 mg at night taken with fluids and to build up the dose if necessary by adding 25–50 mg in the morning, or alternatively long-acting Indocid-R can be taken in a total dose of 75 mg at night.

(d) Naproxen. Nearly as powerful as indomethacin and less likely to have side-effects, it is especially useful in elderly patients.

(e) Mefenamic acid (Ponstan). Some favour this NSAID as it also has a moderate direct analgesic effect.

(f) Phenylbutazone. The first NSAID to be introduced, this is a powerful drug but should be used in moderate doses (100 mg three or four times daily) for only very short periods, or else there is a risk of blood dyscrasia. Small doses (100 mg daily or b.d.) may be safely given for longer periods.

(g) Piroxicam (Feldene). Another useful alternative to indomethacin when this is not tolerated, piroxicam is long acting and needs to be given only once daily (usually 20 mg at night).

SUMMARY: DRUGS IN BACK PAIN

(1) Analgesics, sedatives, muscle relaxants, psychotropic and anti-inflammatory drugs are all useful in backache.

(2)   Analgesics are mild (such as paracetamol), moderately powerful (Panadeine Co.), powerful (buprenorphine) or very powerful (listed drugs such as pethidine).

(3)   The most useful sedatives are tranquillizers such as diazepam or temazepam.

(4)   Tranquillizers such as diazepam also 'double' as muscle relaxants, which are often prescribed together with analgesics.

(5)   Tranquillizers such as diazepam are prescribed in larger doses when anxiety is prominent. It is rarely necessary to use 'major tranquillizers' such as chlorpromazine. Antidepressive drugs such as amitriptyline are required when depression is a factor.

(6)   Non-steroidal anti-inflammatory drugs are useful in acute episodes of spinal osteoarthritis and, in small doses, for some patients with chronic back pain. Phenylbutazone in particular has a powerful, 'specific' effect in ankylosing spondylitis. NSAIDs have little proven effect in acute disc lesions.

References

Crown, S. (1978). Treatment of depression in back pain. *Rheum. Rehabil.*, **17**, 114

Hingorani, K. (1966). Diazepam in backache – a double-blind controlled trial. *Ann. Phys. Med.*, **8**, 303

4
Physiotherapy in Back Pain

Physiotherapy (physical therapy in the USA) is treatment by physical (as opposed to medical) methods. Although it is widely used in the treatment of back pain, unfortunately the correct indications and methods of prescribing physical treatment are poorly understood by many physicians. This responsibility therefore falls on the physiotherapist (physical therapist) who fortunately, by dint of training and experience, is usually able to prescribe the correct treatment. However, is this right – should we expect a pharmacist to prescribe a drug without medical guidance?

This chapter is intended as a guide to the indications for physiotherapy in backache and its practical applications. It is divided into the following sections:

1. THE AIMS OF PHYSIOTHERAPY

In back pain physiotherapy is used to (a) relieve pain, (b) improve the movements of the spine and (c) strengthen the back muscles. Physiotherapists also teach patients 'back discipline' and home exercises (see Chapter 9).

In acute back pain and sciatica, physiotherapy does not play a large part in treatment. It is more important where the acute attack is resolving and in chronic lumbago and sciatica.

Unlike drug treatment, the principles of physical therapy are not taught in most medical schools and so newly-qualified doctors know little or nothing about it. As a result the therapist must be adept at deciding on the correct procedure, but she still should be supplied with a *reasonable diagnosis and basic instructions.* For example, she may be asked to mobilize a stiff spine following a mild disc prolapse. It is not necessary to specify the exact type of treatment (e.g. shortwave diathermy), though rheumatologists and orthopaedic surgeons who are well accustomed to ordering physiotherapy and assessing the results tend to be more specific in the type of therapy requested.

Regarding frequency of therapy, it is customary to request three sessions weekly for 2–4 weeks. However, twice-weekly therapy is sometimes given and this is not ideally efficient. Six to eight treatments (not more than twelve), are usually enough. Continued improvement at the end of a session of treatment is the only sensible reason for extension of treatment. Following exercises or mobilization therapy and sometimes lumbar traction, patients should be taught prophylactic exercises to continue at home (see Chapter 9).

2. 'OPEN' AND 'CLOSED' ACCESS TO PHYSIOTHERAPY DEPARTMENTS

In the United Kingdom it is usual for referral for physiotherapy to be open to medical staff within the hospital only, and not to general practitioners and others wishing to refer cases from 'outside'. Such departments are known as 'closed' and this may be necessary because of inadequacy of physiotherapy staffing, so that it is possible to cope only with internal referrals. It is now becoming more widely accepted that the possibility of referral from without is desirable in many if not most instances. Direct referral from general practitioners leads to a shorter wait for treatment, as there is often considerable delay for an appointment with the consultant, and there is some evidence that this facilitation of early treatment allows patients to return to work more quickly. In 'open access', however, diagnosis is less likely to be accurate and, if the system is poorly controlled, there is a risk that the department could be flooded with inappropriate referrals. The superintendent physiotherapist's role is of paramount importance in this context and it is imperative that she initially assesses every patient eligible for open access physiotherapy. It is also important that the physiotherapist treating the patient should be able to have access to consultant opinion where she deems this necessary.

A short study of 'open access' physiotherapy was carried out in 1982 at Princess Alexandra Hospital, Harlow. Of 65 patients referred, by general practitioners, the superintendent physiotherapist considered

54 (83%) were suitable for treatment. A month after the conclusion of physiotherapy patients and referring doctors were sent questionnaires designed to assess the desirability of 'open access'. The results are summarized in Tables 4.1 and 4.2. It turned out that most patients were in fact those with neck or back pain. Whereas six or seven sessions were usually required, up to 12 sessions were needed in a significant number of patients. Whereas most patients where happy about this arrangement, 25% would have preferred to see a consultant in the first instance, before embarking on physiotherapy. Eventually six

Table 4.1   Survey of open access to physiotherapy

Classifications	Numbers
Total referred/assessed by Supt. Physio.	65
Sexes	
Male	30
Female	35
Ages	
Range	12–70
Median group	50–60
Under 30 y	5
Conditions	
Back, neck pain	42 (65%)
Others	23 (35%)
Diagnosis supplied	48 (75%)
Duration of symptoms	
< 2/52	3
2–4/52	20 (30%)
	Otherwise mostly evenly distributed up to 1 y
> 1 y	16
X-rays available	40 (61%)
Physiotherapy arranged	54 (83%)
Physiotherapy techniques	
Heat-U.S. alone	7
Maitland	16
Traction	23
Exercises taught	10
Hydrotherapy	1
Advice only	5
Number of sessions	
< 6	17
6 (approx.)	16
8–12	19
> 12	2

Table 4.2   Results of open access survey

Classifications	Numbers
1. Recorded by physiotherapist after treatment	
Better ('cured') or nearly	32 (59%)
Moderately improved	15 (28%)
Total satisfactory improvement	47 (87%)
Slight or no improvement	8 (15%)
'Should have seen consultant first'	6
2. Patients' replies to subsequent questionnaire	
Number returned	44 (81%)
Generally satisfied with treatment	42 (78%)
Not satisfied with treatment	12 (22%)
Physiotherapist recorded better or nearly – patient recorded unsatisfied	9
Better after treatment, improvement not maintained at time of questionnaire	10
Off work, back after treatment	14
Patient would have preferred consultant appointment first	13
Subsequent consultant appointment arranged	9
3. GPs' replies to questionnaire	
GPs sent questionnaire	28
Number returned	25
Generally in favour of 'open access'	25
Any problems encountered	0
Happier for patients to see consultant first before physiotherapy ordered	0

patients did in fact get referred for a consultant opinion because they failed to improve with physiotherapy, and the original diagnosis was thought to be incorrect in four of these.

In a further recent study (Ellman *et al.*, 1982), 'open' physiotherapy records were sampled over a 12-month period and compared with similar records of 'closed' referral from the rheumatology outpatient department. Again back and neck pain figured most frequently. 'Open access' referrals were seen within an average of 5 days, as compared with 24 days' wait to see a clinician who then arranged physiotherapy. The waiting time for a rheumatology appointment in fact fell from 50 to 24 days (in the Harlow study only a temporary fall in the waiting-list occurred) and, more significantly, the percentage of rheumatology patients referred for physiotherapy fell from 75% to 45%.

Summarizing, open access by general practitioners to the physiotherapy department in a general hospital is usually desirable. The attitude and control of the superintendent physiotherapist is important. The referring general practitioner has overall responsibility for the case, but the physiotherapist should be able to approach a consultant if she requires any advice.

3. HEAT AND COLD THERAPY

Applications of *heat* are made for their analgesic and muscle-relaxing effect prior to exercise therapy, manipulation or traction. It is a waste of time to use them in isolation: as one patient put it, 'soothing while I was having it, but my back quickly froze up on the trip home!'

Therapeutic heat can be applied to the lumbar spine in several ways – using a radiant heat lamp (Figure 19), shortwave diathermy, microwave diathermy or simply hot moist packs. There is not much to choose between these various modalities. *Shortwave diathermy* (SWD, Figure 20), where a high-frequency current is converted into heat in the tissues, is supposed to penetrate more deeply and so is often prescribed for deeply-situated joints such as the hip. It has been said that SWD 'specifically' relieves osteoarthritic joints (as in lumbar spondylosis) but there is no good evidence for this. *Microwave radiation* (Figure 21) is also converted into heat in the tissues. Both microwave and shortwave diathermy should be avoided whenever there is a

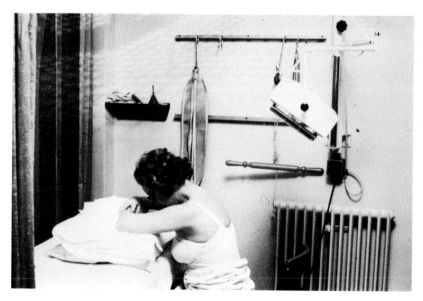

Figure 19 Radiant heat lamp

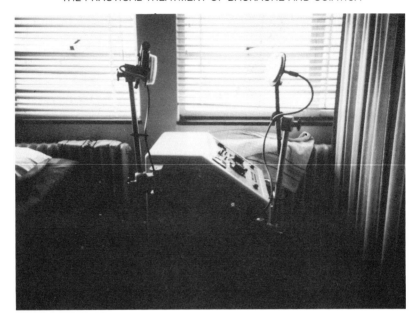

Figure 20 Short-wave diathermy

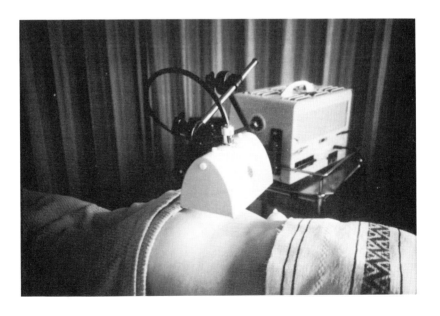

Figure 21 Microwave diathermy

suspicion of either active inflammation of the joints (as in ankylosing spondylitis) or neoplasm.

The application of *ice-packs* or cold compresses can achieve a similar degree of analgesia and muscle relaxation. It is logical to consider cold therapy instead of heat when the patient or the environment is warm and humid, such as on hot summer days.

4. ULTRASOUND THERAPY

Ultrasound (very high-frequency waves using apparatus shown in Figure 22) seems to be particularly useful in treating acute soft-tissue injuries. These are a rare cause of back pain in practice, except on the sports field where minor ligamentous ruptures are said to be respon-

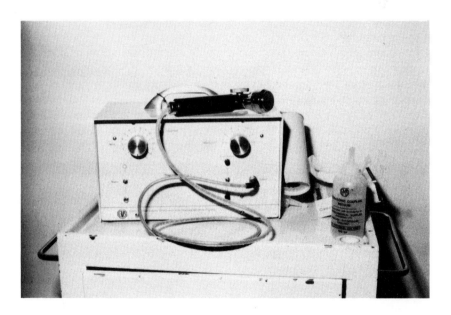

Figure 22 Ultrasound therapy

sible for acute episodes of backache. However, ultrasound generally has a limited place in the treatment of low back pain. It can be used for back pain following a kick at football, where bruising or tearing of a muscle tends to be followed by painful fibrous adhesions. It is also used by some physiotherapists as a method of relaxing painful paravertebral muscle spasm.

5. EXERCISE THERAPY

Back exercises have three functions: (a) *to improve the range of movement*, so enabling more efficient movement in a pain-free range, (b) to *strengthen the paraspinal muscles*, thus achieving a more stable spine and (c) to *improve the posture* generally – as, for example, in preventing and corresting kyphosis. Three types of exercise are prescribed: *extension exercises*, where the back is arched by the action of the extensor muscles (Figure 23) (see Home Exercises, Chapter 9.2); *flexion exercises*, where the back is progressively flexed; and *isometric exercises*, where the muscles are tightened while lying supine but there is no discernible movement of the back. In *'mobilization exercises'* a mixture of the above is used and these are often more easily accomplished in the hydrotherapy pool. Flexion exercises may be hazardous in patients with actual or impending lumbar disc prolapse because they may 'squeeze out' a pathological disc, as shown by the onset (or worsening) of sciatica, so should certainly be avoided in such patients.

In order to mobilize the back, physiotherapists often use certain manipulative techniques known as *Maitland manipulations* (Figure 24) together with exercise therapy. In subsiding or chronic back pain, correct posture is taught, as well as 'back discipline' particularly

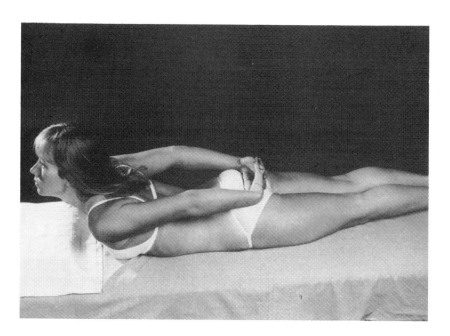

Figure 23 Lumbar exercises: a back extension exercise

related to bending, lifting and carrying. A patient with a acutely painful back should not be expected to carry out exercises which might aggravate or increase pain, though sometimes patients with ankylosing spondylitis find exercises helpful even during relatively acute stages.

Prophylactic back exercises are supposed to prevent future attacks by building an 'internal corset', but in fact it is uncommon for the back muscles to waste. Nevertheless, in recurrent conditions such as lumbar intervertebral joint derangements or mild disc lesions there is no doubt that exercises carried out two or three times daily can reduce the frequency if not the severity of attacks. This is not the case in the hypermobile spine (loose back syndrome) where spinal exercises only stretch ligaments which are already stressed by hypermobility.

6. HYDROTHERAPY

Hydrotherapy means treatment in water and usually indicates exercise therapy carried out in the deep pool. This is a special pool which exists in most hospitals where the water is very warm, being heated to 36 °C, encouraging muscle relaxation so that exercises which the patient would otherwise find difficult or impossible can be attempted. Hydrotherapy is most useful for the wholly stiff and painful back such as in ankylosing spondylitis and in severe cases of spinal

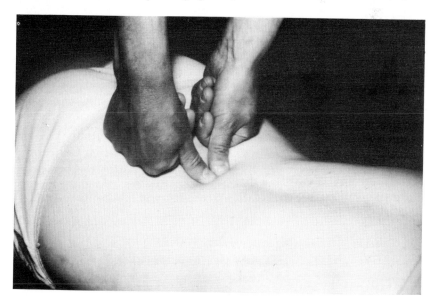

Figure 24 Maitland manipulation of lumbar spine

57

osteoarthritis. By virtue of its buoyancy water allows exercise therapy to take place with gravity removed – that is, it assists active exercises. Alternatively it can be used as a resistance to movement in resisted exercises.

7. LUMBAR TRACTION

There are two types of lumbar traction: (a) intermittent traction, for outpatients with back pain, and (b) continuous (sustained) traction, for the patient in hospital.

In general, *intermittent lumbar traction* is prescribed for back pain syndromes with mild or moderate sciatica or referred pain. Only patients with reasonably mobile spines can tolerate traction, otherwise it may lead to increased spinal pain and muscle spasm. In any event it is desirable to precede traction with 10–15 minutes' local heat (or cold) to the lumbar spine and it may be helpful for the patient to take a muscle-relaxant (such as diazepam 5–10 mg) an hour before commencing treatment. A course of six to ten sessions of lumbar traction often leads to subsidence of sciatica. Traction is put on the pelvis, up to 85 kg force (using weights or mechanical apparatus) for about 30 minutes (Figure 25). Although clinical experience seems to validate the efficacy of traction, it is intriguing that so far there has been no satisfactory controlled trial. Again, how it works is not known – it is said to draw a disc protrusion towards the centre by negative pressure. There is some evidence that traction is less likely to be effective if there is definite neurological deficit in the legs.

Continuous traction for hospitalized patients used to be applied to the legs, but this has been replaced by continuous pelvic traction – claimed to be much less conducive to the development of thrombophlebitis. In acute disc lesions the patient is put to bed with continuous pelvic traction of 15–20 kg, using pulleys and weights (Figure 26). The bed is sometimes slightly inclined in order to increase the pull. This certainly serves to keep the patient still and discourage him from rolling over and it has been said that it is this enforced rest which is therapeutic rather than any significant distraction of the disc! As improvement occurs the weights are gradually decreased and finally the traction is removed, and the patient is gradually mobilized.

SUMMARY; PHYSIOTHERAPY IN BACK PAIN

In back pain, physiotherapy is used to relieve pain (usually prior to exercise therapy), improve spinal movements and strengthen back muscles.

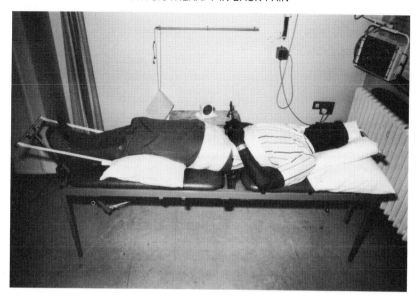

Figure 25   Intermittent lumbar traction (out-patient)

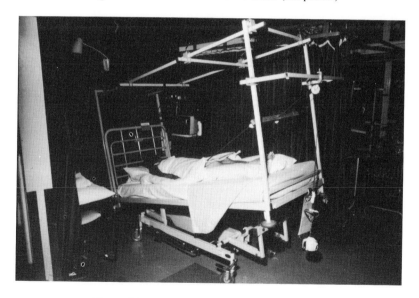

Figure 26   Continuous lumbar traction (in-patient)

Ideally there should be open access to hospital physiotherapy departments for direct referral from general practitioners.

Heat or cold therapy is used for analgesia and muscle-relaxation prior to exercise therapy, manipulation or traction.

Ultrasound is useful in treating soft-tissue lesions of the spine.

Spinal exercises are often combined with manipulative techniques ('Maitland manipulations') to mobilize the spine.

Hydrotherapy allows exercises to take place with gravity removed and with muscular relaxation due to the warm water.

Intermittent lumbar traction is used for treatment of outpatients with sciatica or pain referred to the legs. Continuous pelvic traction is used routinely for patients hospitalized for intervertebral disc lesions.

References

Kendall, P.H. and Jenkins, J.M. (1968). Exercises for backache – a double-blind controlled trial. *Physiotherapy*, **54**, 154

Maitland, G.D. (1977). *Vertebral Manipulation*. 4th Edn. (London: Butterworth)

Nachemson, A. (1969). Physiotherapy for low back pain patients. A critical look. *Scand. J. Rehabil.*, **1**, 85

5
Spinal Manipulation

There is no doubt that spinal manipulation, which is usually carried out without general anaesthesia, is effective in many common varieties of back pain. The general indications for manipulation have been outlined in Chapter 2; in this chapter the indications and techniques are described in more detail.

1. RATIONALE OF MANIPULATION

Manipulation involves forced movements of the spine in various directions with the object of restoring a full and painless range of movements as possible. The following mechanisms of action can operate:

(1) Manipulation can release a joint 'hitch', the internal derangement that results in blocking of certain back movements. It is sometimes possible to show a dramatic and immediate objective improvement in such patients following manipulation.

(2) It can stretch periarticular adhesions in patients whose back trouble has been going on for more than a few weeks. The intervertebral joint is a complex structure including two apophyseal joints as well as the disc 'joint' itself. There is evidence that structures other than the disc, dura mater and nerve roots are involved; for example an epidural injection of local anaesthetic will often relieve the nerve root pain but leave the low back pain, indicating that it has failed to reach structures responsible for the latter. When a patient has been immobilized for some weeks, either in bed or due to painful muscle spasm, the intervertebral joint complex stiffens and

manipulations may be more effective for dealing with this than simple exercieses.

(3) Manipulation can alter the relationship between the disc protrusion and the nerve root in some patients with sciatica.

Manipulation is useless in ligamentous (postural) backache, as the joints move freely already. It is contraindicated in recent central disc herniation (as shown by lumbar kyphosis and bilateral limitation of straight-leg-raising), indeed here it stands a good chance of causing lateral prolapse and changing low back pain into sciatica. Forceful manipulation can be harmful in spondylolisthesis and should be avoided where there is any joint instability. It is often stated that manipulation is very dangerous when there is serious pathology, such as secondary bone tumour. Strangely enough, however, experience has shown that this is rarely the case – vertebrae softened by osteoporosis or secondary deposits do not seem to be 'crushed' by manipulation – indeed, this is far more likely to happen spontaneously when the patient weightbears and exerts his muscles. The one potential disaster from manipulation results from failure to recognize signs of pressure on the cauda equina (see Chapter 2) for, if an incipient root lesion of the second sacral nerve is transformed into a complete palsy, bladder and bowel function may be permanently impaired.

2. INDICATIONS FOR MANIPULATION

The indications are summarized as follows:

(1) *Intervertebral joint derangements.* 'Specific thrust' manipulations (see below) are the best approach.

(2) *Low back pain of any variety with restricted movements* that has continued for more than a few weeks. Here one starts with mobilizing manipulations, these gentler manoeuvres being less likely to cause a temporary exacerbation of pain in such patients. When it has been established that manipulation is being well tolerated, specific thrusts may be added to improve mobilization.

(3) *Some cases of sciatica.* Manipulation is not very very effective in recent sciatica, especially if due to large disc herniations where there is marked diminution of straight-leg-raising (less than 40 °), or if there are objective signs of substantial nerve root pressure such as muscle weakness or widespread numbness and hypoalgesia. However, for sciatica persisting despite adequate bed rest, straight-leg-raising more than 40 ° and only minimal root signs

(such as a small area of numbness and a diminished or even an absent reflex, but no muscle weakness), then it is worthwhile considering manipulation designed to alter the relationship between the disc protrusion and the nerve root. This is often easier and more effective if carried out under the relaxation of a general anaesthetic, when recovery will be initiated in 50–60% patients. It is particularly valuable in the patient who fails to respond to conservative treatment in hospital or who goes on for several months with enough pain to demand active treatment yet has insufficient root signs to justify a radiculogram or, if a radiculogram is carried out, no definite disc protrusion can be identified.

3. MANIPULATION TECHNIQUES

There are two basic types of manipulation: 'mobilizing manipulations' and 'specific thrusts'. Others are the 'sciatic nerve stretch' and the 'lumbar vertical lift'.

Mobilizing manipulations

These are passive movements done repetitively and aimed at coaxing a progressively greater range of spinal movement as the patient relaxes. Mobilizing manipulations take more time than 'specific thrusts and are therefore suitable for delegation to physiotherapists, who usually carry out the movements described by G. Maitland ('Maitland manipulations'). Such manoeuvres are particularly beneficial in patients left with a stiff and painful back after the acute muscle spasm has subsided. This technique is safe even in the presence of quite marked degenerative changes. A course of Maitland manipulations is often followed by showing the patient a set of back exercises which he can continue to do at home.

Specific thrust manipulations

One sudden movement is used to move a spinal joint, which usually responds by a 'click' or 'pop' as the joint seal releases. The aim is to move one particular segment of the spine. To do this the slack is taken up below and above the joint, then an additional sudden thrust of high velocity but low amplitude is imparted to it. Ideally, one tries to make the thrust quick though with only a small increase in the range of movement, as if the thrust is made over a large range of movement the ligaments and capsules of the apophyseal joints and possibly the

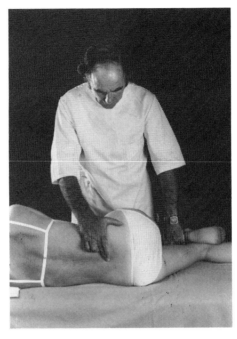

Figure 27a Lumbar rotational manipulation: (a) the top leg is flexed until tension is felt at the inter-spinous ligaments

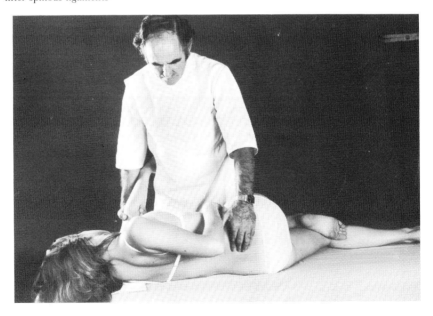

Figure 27b Lumbar rotational manipulation: (b) the lower arm is drawn forward until rotation of the spine is felt down to the segment

annulus of the disc joint will be strained, with subsequent exacerbation of symptoms.

The most useful specific thrust is the *rotational technique*. As already mentioned, this is contraindicated in recent central disc herniations. The patient is positioned lying on one side and the top leg flexed until tension is felt at the interspinous ligaments of the segment one wishes to mobilize (Figure 27). The lower arm is drawn forwards until rotation of the upper spine is felt to reach down to the same segment. At this point the two levers are maintained by the doctor pressing in opposite directions with his two arms and a small sharp additional thrust is given (Figure 28). Although this manipulation is basically rotational, the patient's position can be arranged so that the lumbar spine is in flexion or extension – a good guiding rule is to place the patient in the position which is most comfortable for him. For example, if a patient is unable to fully backward bend but has a reasonable range of forward bending, then the manipulation is best done with the lumbar spine in slight flexion.

The sciatic nerve stretch

For some time it has been recognized that stretching the sciatic nerve

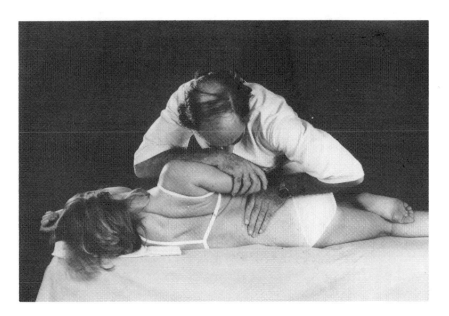

Figure 28 Lumbar rotational manipulation: (c) the two levers are maintained by the doctor pressing in opposite directions and a small additional thrust given

by doing a 'forced straight-leg-raising test' under general anaesthesia can be useful in sciatica. This is more effective if carried out in combination with a rotational manipulation of the lumbar spine: the patient is arranged with the painful leg uppermost, the physician straddles the leg so that the straight leg is brought up to the point of limitation noted at examination, then this is brought further simultaneously with a lumbar rotational manipulation.

The lumbar vertical lift

This is a very safe technique, which can be used even where there is central disc herniation. It is best done with the patient standing back to back with the doctor who usually stands on a small raised platform (Figure 29). By bending and straightening the knees, the physician

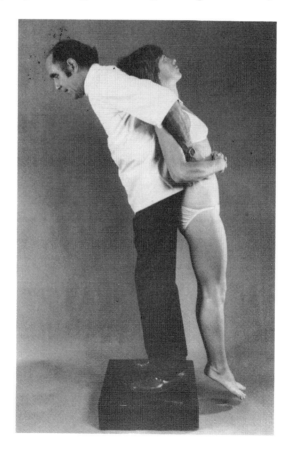

Figure 29 The lumbar vertical lift

imparts gentle oscillations to the lumbar spine and then, by suddenly straightening against the oscillation, imparts a vertical thrust. A successful vertical lift manipulation is often accompanied by a soft click and immediate relief of symptoms. Should backward bending be blocked or cause sharp pain, then this manoeuvre cannot be done standing and the sitting position is used.

SUMMARY

(1) Manipulation acts by releasing an intervertebral joint derangement, stretching periarticular adhesions or altering the disc protrusion/nerve root relationship in sciatica.

(2) Manipulation is indicated for intervertebral joint derangements, persisting low back pain with restricted movements, persisting sciatica due to small disc lesions.

(3) Manipulation is not indicated in ligamentous backache, central disc herniation and the cauda equina syndrome.

(4) The two main types of spinal manipulation are 'mobilizing manipulations' (including Maitland manipulations carried out by physiotherapists) and 'specific thrusts'. Other methods include the 'sciatic nerve stretch' and the 'lumbar vertical lift'.

References

Doran, D.M.L. and Newell, D.J. (1975). Manipulation in treatment of low back pain in multi-centre study. *Br. Med. J.*, **2**, 161

Maitland, G.D. (1977). *Vertebral Manipulation*. 4th Edn. (London; Butterworth)

Mathews, J.A. and Yates, D.A.H. (1969). Reduction of lumbar disc prolapse by manipulation. *Br. Med. J.*, **3**, 696

Sims-Williams, H., Jayson, M.I.V., Young, S.M.S., Baddeley, H. and Collins, E. (1978). Controlled trial of mobilization and manipulation for patients with low back pain in general practice. *Br. Med. J.*, **2**, 1338

6
Injection Techniques

Local steroid injections, sclerosing injections and epidural injections all have a place in the treatment of back pain and sciatica. The advent of hydrocortisone injections revolutionized the treatment of many common ligamentous and tendon lesions, such as supraspinatus tendinitis, but they are less commonly employed in back pain. They can be effective in strains of the lumbar spine, the problem being to identify correctly the soft tissues at fault, then to place the steroid successfully. Where the spinal ligaments are chronically overstretched (as in the hypermobility syndrome) steroid injections are less effective and better results are obtained from sclerosing injections.

1. LOCAL STEROID INJECTIONS

Local steroid injections are useful for:

(1) Acute ligamentous strains of the supraspinous, interspinous and sacro-iliac ligaments, often after sports or other injury.

(2) Apophyseal joint strains giving rise to a synovitis, often on a background of formerly asymptomatic osteoarthritis of the apophyseal joints.

Some advocate injections of 'trigger points' in the paravertebral muscles with steroid. Bourne (1979) suggests that in such cases pain is due to irritation of pain-receptor nerve endings by oedematous muscle fibres which stretch and becomes less oedamatous when injected by triamcinolone acetonide owing to its fibrinolytic action, and claims statistically superior results when compared with patients injected with xylocaine only. This raises the whole dubious question of 'fibrositis', which has been purposely omitted in this book as it is not generally accepted that chemical abnormalities of paravertebral muscle are responsible for back pain – rather it is the concept of muscle spasm with which we are most concerned, and in this context it would be thought that trigger points are better treated using acupuncture techniques (see Chapter 7) than steroid injections.

Back pain due to *ligamentous strains or sprains*, often due to a sports injury, is characterized by local tenderness with a full or nearly full range of lumbar movements but pain at the extremes of the range. Infiltration of the ligaments at fault with local anaesthetic should temporarily abolish this pain on movement, and this is then followed by infiltration with local steroid. Pain felt over the sacro-iliac joints may occur in disc prolapses but there is usually no significant tenderness. Marked tenderness of the posterior sacro-iliac ligaments frequently indicates a strain of these ligaments, either in isolation or accompanying a disc lesion, and a local steroid injection may bring a surprising degree of relief. In simple ligamentous strains there is no history of sudden 'locking' of the spine, or acute paralysing pain on minor movements, that characterizes acute intervertebral joint derangements and disc herniations. The supraspinous and interspinous ligaments are tested by asking the patient to forward-bend fully; occasionally the ligaments are so sensitive that backward bending also causes pain. The posterior sacro-iliac ligaments can be put on stretch by flexing and adducting the hip joint forcibly. (*Note*: sacro-iliac testing by springing, gapping or compression (see Chapter 1.3) does not usually put sufficient tension on these ligaments to evoke pain.)

As regards steroid injections for *apophyseal joint strains*, the apophyseal (posterior facet) joints are true synovial joints and are therefore subject to osteoarthritis and, just as in osteoarthritis of the knee, superimposed strains of these joints may evoke a painful synovitis. Also, consequent enlargement of these joints leads to narrowing of the lateral recesses of the spinal canal and may give rise to pressure on emerging nerve roots. Just as painful synovitis secondary to osteoarthritis of the knee may be resolved by a steroidal injection, recent sprains of the apophyseal joints can be successfully treated in this way. A needle 2 inches (5 cm) long (3 inches (7.5 cm) in the obese) is inserted at a point half an inch (13 mm) from the midline and at the level of the interspace between two spinous processes (Figure 30). The injection of steroid with 2% xylocaine is given in three parts: (a) the needle is introduced vertically downwards until it strikes bone and the first 0.5 ml is injected, (b) the needle is withdrawn an inch (2.5 cm) and angled towards the direction of the head and advanced until bone is reached again, when a further 0.5 ml is injected, and (c) the needle is angled towards the direction of the feet and the third portion of the injection given. By 'fanning out' the injection in this way there is a greater chance of enough material reaching the affected apophyseal joint. However, even if the joint is

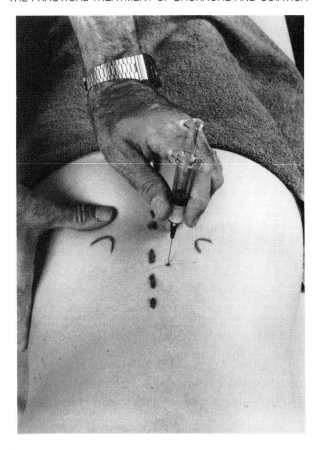

Figure 30   The surface marking position for injecting the left lumbo-sacral apophyseal joint

not actually penetrated, the injection is often effective if the capsule and adjoining ligaments are infiltrated. Clues to which apophyseal joint or joints are at fault are given by local tenderness to the side of the midline and evidence of degenerative changes in the facet joint seen in X-rays taken in the antero-posterior and oblique views.

2. EPIDURAL INJECTIONS

While there is no doubt that epidural injections of dilute local anaesthetic, often with the addition of steroid, are very useful in certain cases of sciatica, the mode of action is not understood. The following is one explanation of their action. When the dural sleeve of a lumbar nerve root is pressed on by a disc protrusion, the resulting pain arises for two reasons: firstly, if the disc protrusion is of any appreciable size the nerve root is stretched over it and pain can arise from the mechanical tension on the nerve; secondly, the root-sleeve becomes slightly red and swollen (as can be seen during disc surgery) indicating a mild degree of inflammation. It is probably the inflammatory factor which is alleviated by epidural injections of a local anaesthetic/steroid mixture. However, others believe that the effect is simply mechanical, the nerve root being separated from the disc by the large volume of fluid.

Epidural injections have a better chance of success where there is a small irritable disc lesion rather than a large protrusion which gives rise to marked reduction of straight leg raising and distinct neurological signs. Generally speaking they are not likely to be successful when the SLR is less than 45°. Also, patients with a moderate-sized protrusion giving sciatica which partly responds to bed rest but leaves residual leg pain persisting for many weeks may also be helped at this later stage by an epidural injection.

The epidural space is the loose space filled with areolar and fatty tissue outside the dura. Epidural injections can be given caudally via the sacral hiatus (the sacral route) or via the L_{3-4} interspace (lumbar route). Contrast medium studies show that the sacral route is the better approach for disc lesions at the lumbosacral level and that the lumbar route is better for the less common, higher L_{3-4} disc lesions. The L_{4-5} space is reached equally well by both approaches. Caudal epidurals have the extra advantage in that the injection is a minor procedure which can be carried out in the course of an ordinary outpatient clinic, a lumbar epidural being a more complicated procedure carrying with it the risk of inadvertent lumbar puncture.

For *caudal epidural injections* in patients of normal build a needle (23 g × 1¼ inches (3 cm) can be used – it is not necessary to use a large-bore, angulated epidural needle. The sacral hiatus is palpated (approximately three fingers below the posterior iliac spines, see Figure 31) and, after the skin has been cleaned with antiseptic, the needle connected to a small syringe containing 1 ml of 1% lignocaine is introduced through the covering ligament. The local anaesthetic is useful as it may be necessary to probe around to find the hiatus, and at the correct site the needle is felt to 'give' as it goes through the ligament. This, and the free flow once in the epidural space, are the best indications of correct insertion and there is no need to advance the needle up the sacral canal. If a vein has been entered, blood enters the syringe and the tip of the needle must be moved until it is clear of the blood vessel. The needle is left *in situ* whilst the syringe is removed and replaced with one containing 20 ml of 0.5% lignocaine in normal saline to which has been added 5 ml of steroid (hydrocortisone, methylprednisolone or triamcinolone – this has been shown to improve chances of

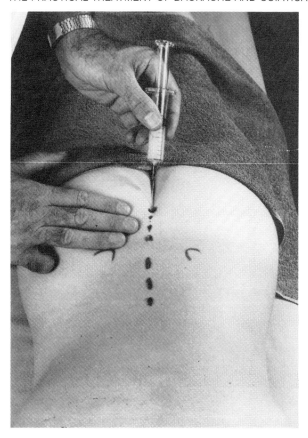

Figure 31 The sacral hiatus is approximately three fingers' breadth below the posterior iliac spines

success – see Yates, 1978). The injection is given very slowly (5 ml/min). Often a twinge of sciatic pain is induced when the solution contacts the sensitive nerve root; after a pause to allow the pain to subside, a further 1 or 2 ml are injected and the needle removed. Gravity does not affect the spread of fluid in the epidural space so the patient can be turned onto his back immediately after the procedure. Straight-leg-raising is then reassessed – if improved, this often, though not invariably, indicates a successful procedure. Some believe that the result is enhanced if the leg raising is forcibly stretched for a moment or two at this stage. After the anaesthetic effect has worn off, up to a week may elapse before improvement starts. It may be necessary to repeat the injection once or even twice to achieve the full benefit, but often there is adequate improvement after a single injection. When entering by the *lumbar route*, a winged lumbar puncture needle with a flat bevel is used and strict asepsis, as for lumbar puncture, is essential. With the patient lying on the side the 3rd–4th lumbar interspace is identified and a skin wheal raised with local anaesthetic. The needle is then introduced and as it approaches the spinal canal a second syringe filled with normal saline is used to produce a hanging drop on the end of the lumbar needle. As the needle is advanced the patient is asked to breathe in and, when the epidural space is entered, the hanging drop is suddenly sucked into the needle. A syringe containing 20 ml of normal saline to which have been added 2–5 ml of steroid is connected and there should be no resistance to the injection which is given rapidly. Normal saline rather than dilute local anaesthetic is always used in the lumbar route because of the possibility of circulatory collapse owing to inadvertent intravascular or intrathecal injection of local anaesthetic.

3. SCLEROSING INJECTIONS

Sclerosing injections for back pain were first introduced by Hackett in 1957. Although (like every enthusiastic innovator) he recommended their use too widely and claimed undue success, it is now felt that there is a place for sclerosing injections in two particular situations:

(1) Intervertebral joint derangements which recur so frequently in

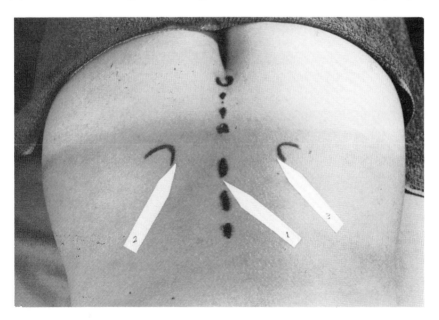

Figure 32 Sclerosing injections are given at three sites (1) the inter-spinous ligaments, (2 & 3) the posterior sacro-iliac ligaments

spite of prophylactic exercises, corsetting etc that another preventive step has to be taken.

(2)   Chronic ligamentous (postural) backache (see Chapter 2).

Sclerosing injections are always given in conjunction with a temporary corset, muscle strengthening exercises and general advice on correct posture and lifting techniques. The material injected consists of 5 ml of 1% xylocaine to which has been added 1 ml of ethanotamine oleate, a substance often used for sclerosing varicose veins. The technique is to infiltrate at three sites – the ligamentous – periosteal junctions of the supraspinous, iliolumbar and (if indicated) posterior sacro-iliac ligaments, 0.5 ml being injected at each point where the ligament is inserted into bone (see Figure 32). Following the injections the patient is warned that there may be increased pain for 1–2 days. The injections are repeated on two more occasions at approximately fortnightly intervals. Improvement may be expected to take place over 3 months.

SUMMARY: INJECTIONS FOR BACKACHE

Local steroid injections may be used for backache due to acute ligamentous strains or apophyseal joint strains.

Caudal epidural injections are useful for mild cases of sciatica where straight-leg-raising is not reduced below 45°, and for residual sciatica following complete bed rest. High lumbar lesions are more effectively treated with lumbar epidurals.

Sclerosing injections are occasionally helpful in recurrent intervertebral joint derangements and in chronic ligamentous backache.

References

Beliveau, P. (1971). A comparison between epidural anaesthesia with and without steroid in the treatment of sciatica. *Rheum. Phys. Med.*, **11**, 40

Bourne, I.H.J. (1979). Treatment of backache with local injections. *Practitioner*, **222**, 708

Hackett, J.S. (1957). *Joint Ligament Relaxation*. (Springfield: Thomas)

Yates, D.W. (1978). A comparison of the types of epidural injection commonly used in the treatment of low back pain and sciatica. *Rheum. Rehabil.*, **17**, 181

7
Acupuncture and Transcutaneous Electrical Nerve Stimulation (TENS)

Acupuncture is often advocated for the relief of pain arising in musculoskeletal structures. Fine needles are inserted into the skin and subcutaneous tissue, sometimes to the periosteum (a particularly sensitive tissue) in order to produce a slightly painful sensory stimulus. If the treatment is successful the original pain is relieved or ameliorated, but how acupuncture works is still unknown. Neither the so-called 'nervous' nor the 'chemical' concept (release of endorphins and encephalins) accounts for the phenomena observed – such as why there is often an interval of days or longer before the beneficial effect is observed, and how and why pain-relief can be so long-lasting. In fact there seems little doubt that acupuncture has a place (admittedly poorly defined) in the treatment of some cases of backache and sciatica.

To date no controlled clinical trial has shown that acupuncture is truly effective. Reported success rates range from 50% (only 5–10% more than the recognized placebo response) to as much as 70%. Again, there is no agreement as to whether it is essential that points on the classical Chinese 'meridians' are stimulated: one trial showed no significant difference between patients having 'true' acupuncture using the classical points and those having 'sham' acupuncture using areas distal from these points. In patients who appear to respond it is not known how much of the beneficial effect is 'real' and how much due to suggestion, i.e. a placebo reaction. All forms of pain-relief treatment – drugs, physiotherapy, or whatever – induce a certain placebo reaction which varies greatly from patient to patient and occurs in as many as 45% cases. On the other hand, it would seem that obviously-suggestible (or 'neurotic') patients who are treated with acupuncture do not necessarily have a greater placebo effect and consequently a better total response. The difference between a 'pure' placebo effect and truly successful acupunture is illustrated by the fact that a placebo effect is normally short-lived whereas acupuncture can give relief lasting weeks, months or even longer. Relief for only a few days after the first acupuncture session probably represents a placebo reaction and does not imply that the treatment will be successful. It should be noted that the placebo effect itself is known to be mediated by release of endorphins and can be blocked by naloxone, just as is thought to be the case with acupuncture. The whole matter is confused, and in the light of today's ignorance the writers make no apology for not attempting to clarify these issues.

Acupuncture and transcutaneous nerve stimulation as used in the treatment of back pain will be described under the following headings:

(In Section (6) a description is given of percutaneous radio frequency denervation).

1. ACUPUNCTURE PROCEDURE

While it is has been pointed out that acupuncture may be effective on applying a sensory stimulus to the skin, there seems little doubt that the efficacy is increased by choosing points to stimulate – usually classical acupuncture points (on the 'meridians') or else areas of increased skin or muscle hypersensitivity. It is now felt that stimulation of such 'trigger areas' is at least effective as using classical points – in one study a 70% correspondence of trigger points and 'classical' points was shown. The practised finger detects small areas of muscle spasm which may or may not be tender to the touch. Lying principally in the paraspinal muscles, these are thought to have low electrical resistance (high conductivity) and they lie over proprioceptive-rich areas such as musculo-tendinous junctions. Stimulation is by inserting thin atraumatic needles which are either left *in situ* for up to 30 minutes or rotated for 30–60 seconds and removed and used for stimulating points one at a time. The discomfort experienced by needling is variable, but the stimulus must be felt by the patient and should be a little painful. Occasionally there is a feeling of numbness and heaviness after stimulation (known by the Chinese as the 'Te Ch'i effect'). The stimulus can be increased by twirling the needle, by inserting it deeper into the tissues or by stimulating the periosteum of an adjacent bony structure, such as the laminae of vertebrae. Sometimes a low-frequency electrical current is used instead of needling. The patient may feel pain radiating outward from the needle; sometimes this radiates up or down the limb and it is interesting that the radiation may correspond to the line of certain meridians. Immediate relief of pain may occur but usually there is a latent period of 4–7 days, sometimes longer, before pain-relief is observed. The patient should be asked *not to judge the effect for a week* and, if treatment has been successful, relief continues for at least another few days. Acupuncture is then repeated and third and fourth treatments, should they be necessary, can be given at successive 3 or 4-weekly intervals.

2. ACUPUNCTURE THEORY

As already mentioned, it is still unclear how acupuncture achieves its effect. It is thought that stimulation of 'acupuncture points' by needle insertion relieves pain by one or both of the following mechanisms.

(1) The Neural Mechanism, through the gate control of the spinal cord. Acupuncture activates receptors from which impulses are sent. Impulses sent through the large myelinated (A delta) sensory nerves (which transmit 'fast pain') cut off noxious pain impulses travelling through small unmyelinated C fibres transmitting 'slow pain', including all forms of pathological pain, at the substantia gelatinosa in the posterior horn of the grey matter. However, there is increasing evidence that acupuncture principally activates the descending inhibitory pathways from the reticular formation and other areas of the brain to the spinal cord. The afferents may also synapse on substantia gelatinosa cells and produce segmental analgesia by release of encephalins.

(2) The Chemical Mechanism, by release of encephalins and endorphins – the 'physiological opiates' – from neurons of the periaqueductal grey matter, which perhaps combine with opiate receptors in midbrain structures and activate the dorsolateral funiculus to inhibit nociceptive neurons in lamina areas 1–6 of the substantia gelatinosa of the posterior horn. It has been shown

that c.s.f. concentrations of the opiate-like peptides β-endorphin and met-encephalin which are low before treatment rise after acupuncture.

The classical acupuncture points as described by the Chinese lie on 'meridians' which, though quite unanatomical, as already mentioned may indicate the distribution of pain referred from a stimulated area. Fourteen meridians are described, each being identified by the name of an organ (e.g. bladder, spleen) though this is purely a question of nomenclature.

3. ACUPUNCTURE POINTS IN BACK PAIN AND SCIATICA

The main *classical points* to be stimulated in back pain and sciatica are principally 'bladder points':

Lumbar spine:
    Paravertebral tender areas ('Luatno-chiachi' points)
    Bladder 31–34 (over sacral foraminae)

Sacro-iliac joints:
    Bladder 26 (over 'dimples' of sacro-iliac joints)

Legs:
    Bladder 60 (lateral malleolus)
    Bladder 56 (mid-calf)
    Gallbladder 34 (medial to head of fibula)
    Bladder 54 (or 40) (lower boundary of popliteal fossa)
    Bladder 51 (midpoint of central posterior thigh)

In addition to the classical points, tender points or areas of spasm of the paravertebral and other musculature of the back lying in the vicinity of or adjacent to the lesion may be stimulated. It is possible to adopt a somewhat anatomical approach to needling when pain and tenderness are referred from the lumbar spine: if they are referred in the S_1 distribution, the back of the calf and lateral malleolus are needled; if they are referred from the upper lumbar spine, points on the front of the thigh and leg are needled.

4. INDICATIONS FOR ACUPUNCTURE IN BACK PAIN AND SCIATICA

It is not unusual for acupuncture to be the preferred first line of treatment in backache and sciatica. Used by physicians, however, it is more useful, as an adjunct to more standard treatments, such as manipulation and physiotherapy. Used in conjunction with these, acupuncture may relieve residual pain, especially where this is referred and where there are corresponding tender points.

To summarize, acupuncture may be useful in low back pain as follows.

(1) Where pain is *referred* across the back to buttocks, hips or legs. (Referred pain must be distinguished from root (sciatic) pain due to impingement of a disc or osteophyte on a nerve root, usually more severe than referred pain – this is rarely relieved by acupuncture.)

(2) In *chronic low back pain,* especially where this is relieved by walking and aggravated by immobility – (i.e. associated with osteoarthritis).

(3) In *residual pain* following manipulation or physiotherapy.

(4) Where *muscle spasm* is prominent and an important factor in producing back pain.

(5) In some cases of *ligamentous backache,* as seen in the hypermobility (loose back) syndrome (see Chapter 2) – sometimes acupuncture is the only way of relieving back pain in this condition.

On the other hand, acupuncture is usually ineffective in cases of severe back pain or sciatica, when the pain arises from pathological bone conditions, or when there are prominent psychological factors influencing the symptoms. *It must be stressed that acupuncture is never helpful in purely psychogenic backache, even though it is often mistakenly suggested for patients with this condition.*

5. TRANSCUTANEOUS NERVE STIMULATION (TENS) IN BACK PAIN

Transcutaneous nerve stimulation (TENS or TNS) is high-frequency (usually 50–150 Hz) sensory stimulation using pulsed, usually square-wave or biphasic current. The small 9 volt battery-operated machine is strapped to the patient and the conductive electrodes attached to either the painful area or tender points detected in a similar manner to acupuncture points. Usually one electrode is placed centrally (e.g. over a tender paravertebral area), the other over a distal tender point on the leg. The intensity, the pulse frequency and sometimes the wave-form can be individually controlled, by either the physician or physiotherapist initially trying the treatment and finding the optimum points, intensity and frequency, then by the patient who takes the machine home and operates it himself. Treatments should last at least 30 minutes, perhaps an hour, and patients may use TENS daily, twice daily or more often. In backache, ideally the frequency of treatments can gradually be reduced until it is no longer required.

Unlike acupuncture, which (as has been pointed out) is low-frequency stimulation, TENS is more often effective in severe sciatica, occasionally even the intractable type often associated with arachnoiditis or nerve root fibrosis which can complicate previous laminectomy.

6. PERCUTANEOUS RADIOFREQUENCY FACET DENERVATION

This is not a form of acupuncture or TENS, but another pain-relief technique which can be effective in patients with intractable backache. It is included briefly in this chapter for convenience.

Formerly rhizolysis – cutting the small sensory nerve supplying the intervertebral facet-joints – was carried out to relieve pain arising from osteoarthritis of these joints. This procedure is largely giving way to burning or freezing the posterior primary rami of these nerves. In percutaneous radiofrequency denervation the electrode is guided by using the image intensifier, the tissues around its tip are heated and the required lesion produced. In cryoanalgesic techniques the nerves are destroyed by cooling the probe to temperatures around $-70\,°C$.

SUMMARY

Acupuncture by needle stimulation can be useful in mild cases of back pain, particularly when the pain is referred, when it is relieved by walking and aggravated by immobility, when residual pain follows manipulation or physiotherapy and where there is prominent muscle spasm. Under modern ('Western') techniques, localized areas of muscle spasm and tenderness are stimulated, rather than the numerous points located on the classical Chinese meridians.

Transcutaneous nerve stimulation (TENS) is a form of self-administered high-frequency stimulation which is useful in relieving some cases of severe sciatica.

Percutaneous radiofrequency facet denervation and cryoanalgesia can be useful for a small number of patients with intractable pain arising from one or a few osteoarthritic apophyseal (facet) joints.

References

Fox, E.J. and Melzack, R. (1976). Transcutaneous electrical stimulation and acupuncture: comparison of treatment in low back pain. *Pain*, **2**, 141

Shealy, C.N. (1975). Percutaneous radiofrequency denervation of spinal facets in back pain. *J. Neurosurg.*, **43**, 448

8
Adjuncts to the Conservative Treatment of Backache

1. AGGRAVATING FACTORS

In assessing a patient with back pain it is important to note carefully any *precipating and aggravating factors*. Injury is of course the commonest factor precipitating disc or intervertebral joint lesions and this may vary from obvious severe trauma, such as falling onto the back from a height, to minor events such as a twist at work or simply bending down and lifting a light object. Such precipitating factors may initiate back pain in a patient with some predisposing underlying disorder of the spine, such as osteoarthritis, lumbar instability, spondylolysis or spondylolisthesis.

Of great importance in the assessment and treatment of backache are aggravating factors, extraspinal conditions which increase back pain. Examples of important aggravating factors are as follows.

(1) Psychological disorders – principally anxiety, depression, secondary gain and malingering. These are discussed in Chapter 1.5.

(2) Occupational factors. Back pain is often closely associated with the patient's work, particularly when bending and lifting are implicated. Sometimes recurrent twisting movements are required and this is equally stressful on the spine, particularly if twisting is combined with lifting in one movement.

(3) Recreational factors. Various games, sports and physical exercise may aggravate a back syndrome. It may be less obvious that yoga and similar activities often include harmful movements conducive to back pain.

(4) Postural abnormalities of the legs. Important examples are inequality of leg-lengths, genu valgum or varum and pes planus. These throw a mechanical strain on the spine and should be corrected wherever possible. In women, high heels and 'platform shoes' often cause trouble by tilting the pelvis, so exaggerating lumbar lordosis.

(5) Hormonal factors. Various endocrine disorders may aggravate backache. *Hypothyroidism*, often not clinically obvious, can cause stiffness and pain in the paravertebral muscles just as in muscles elsewhere. (Sometimes this becomes apparent when, during the clinical examinations, sustained relaxation of the ankle-jerks is noted). It is confirmed by measuring the T_3, T_4 and TSH. *Premenstrual tension* often causes backache and, of course, lumbar discomfort in the first few days of the *menstrual period* is well known. The backache of *pregnancy*, usually coming on at about the fifth month, is said to be due to softening of the sacro-iliac ligaments which are exposed to strain inflicted by the enlarging uterus and developing fetus. As well as this, lumbar disc lesions are common in late pregnancy. Backache often becomes apparent at the *menopause*, probably due to exacerbations of lumbar spondylosis which flares up at this time (as does osteoarthritis elsewhere). *Postmenopausal backache* due to osteoporosis is a well-known entity due to drain of calcium from the bones and marked loss of calcium can lead to crush fractures of the vertebrae.

(6) Sexual intercourse. This may aggravate backache in both men and women. Also, successful treatment of a lumbar lesion (as for example by manipulation) not infrequently leads to improved sexual performance and satisfaction!

(7) Gynaecological disorders. Contrary to what used to be believed, it is very unusual for genito-urinary lesions to be a primary cause of backache. However, this often follows the *sustained lithotomy position* used in gynaecological operations; and certain infections, such as a chronic cervical erosion, salpingitis or recurrent urinary infection, may doubtedly aggravate pre-existing backache. Recent work suggests that such infective foci can also be associated with certain cases of sacro-iliitis and ankylosing spondylitis in women (De Roo, 1978; Golding, 1982). While

spondylitis is nearly always associated with the histocompatibility antigen HLA–B27, mild cases of sacro-iliitis in females may be B27-negative and associated with subclinical genitourinary infection. In such cases the sacro-iliac joints, while appearing normal on the plain X-ray, may appear 'hot' when scanned by bone-seeking isotopes.

2. SUPPORTING THE BACK: CORSETS AND BRACES

Lumbar supports have *four functions:*

(1) To provide temporary *support* (both physical and psychological) in patients with acute backache,

(2) To *prevent or minimize spinal movements* in chronic lumbar disorders such as spondylosis,

(3) To *'splint or stabilize* one or more areas of the spine where there is evidence of instability, as in spondylolisthesis or spondylolysis,

(4) As a prophylactic measure, to *prevent recurrence* of back pain in patients liable to back strain for occupational reasons.

Most patients with low back pain can do without corsetting and so *lumbar supports should not be routinely prescribed.* A corset is indicated only when one of the above indications is clearly present, and the reason for the corset should always be explained to the patient. A temporary support should be returned as soon as the acute lumbago has subsided. Another use of a temporary support is as a trial measure in lumbar spondylosis where there has been poor response to other treatment; if it is effective, the temporary support is replaced by a more substantial permanent corset.

Some form of support, usually a substantial brace (such as the 'Goldthwaite' variety), is nearly always necessary for backache associated with 'weak areas' as in spondylolysis, spondylolisthesis or retrospondylolisthesis, though it is claimed that a belt can sometimes be replaced by an 'internal support' provided by sclerosing injections (see Chapter 6).

There are many varieties of lumbar corset, ranging from the 'temporary' ready-made lumbosacral belts (Figure 33), which are lightweight and often fastened by Velcro, to more rigid corsets fashioned around a steel loop and made to measure, of which the Goldthwaite support is one example. One golden rule applies to every corset: it must *fit properly* and be *comfortable.* Patients only too often are persuaded by the fitter that the corset is satisfactory and attempt to

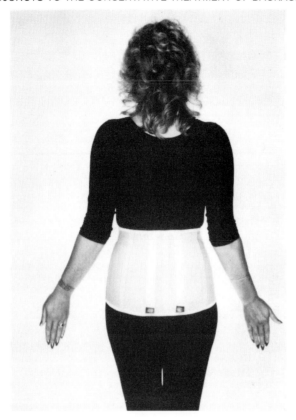

Figure 33 Small (temporary) lumbar support

wear it even though it 'digs in' or 'rides up' the spine. They must be carefully instructed not to accept a belt which does not fit properly, or is
otherwise uncomfortable, but to hand it back to the fitter who should
alter the fitting or, if necessary, try an alternative type of belt –
otherwise it will certainly not be worn, or else will do no good even if
an effort is made to put up with it! The heavy braces of former years
are no longer seen. An exception is the 'extension' brace required
to immobilize the thoracic spine in cases of severe thoracic or
thoraco-lumbar lesions resistant to treatment, where the brace must
extend up between the shoulder-blades and, in the case of high thoracic
lesions (above T_7) shoulderstraps are required to keep the brace snugly
in place (Figure 34).

3. CHAIRS, CAR SEATS AND BEDS

Patients with back problems should be taught to sit straight up and

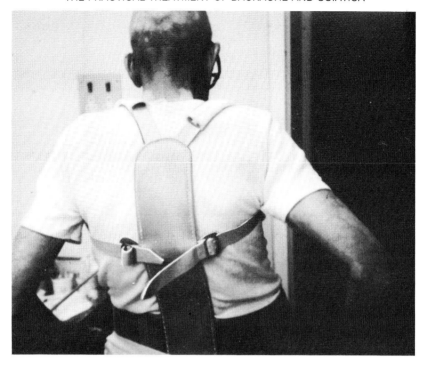

Figure 34 Lumbar brace throracic extension

not to sag in their chair. A chair with a *vertical back* is best and low armchairs should be avoided. Office chairs are often faulty in this respect. Regarding car seats, the degree of lumbar support is very important – it is helpful to put a small cushion in the small of the back as a lumbar support, if this is not already built into the seat-back as is the case in some cars.

A firm mattress is usually advised to give the most comfort in bed, but it is important that the *base under the mattress* is firm. While many patients find it helpful to put a board under the mattress, it should be pointed out that this is not always a help, and it is a question of trial and error. The best sleeping positions are either flat on the back, on one or other side with the hips and knees slightly bent, or flat on the stomach. Whatever position is initially adopted, frequent turning always occurs during sleep and this may be painful where there is a back lesion – turning on a sagging bed is more difficult and painful than turning on a firm bed. Patients with sciatica often adopt a flexed position of the spine and find a cushion under the knee on the affected side gives relief.

SUMMARY

(1) Factors aggravating back pain, which should be corrected if possible, include psychological disorders; strain on the back at work or recreation; postural abnormalities of the legs and feet; hormonal factors such as hypothyroidism and pregnancy; intercourse; and some gynaecological disorders.

(2) Some patients need lumbar supports – for temporary use in acute backache, or to splint the spine in chronic disorders, or to stabilize 'weak' areas such as spondylolisthesis, or to prevent back injury where there is exposure to strain, as in work or gardening. It is imperative that corsets fit exactly and that they are totally acceptable to the patient.

(3) Chairs must have an upright back-rest. A lumbar cushion should be used where a car seat is badly designed.

(4) A firm mattress is often,though not always, desirable for patients with low back pain, and trial-and-error is always required.

References

Anderson, J.A. (1980). Back pain and occupation. In Jayson, M. (ed.). *The Lumbar Spine and Back Pain*. 2nd Edn. (London: Pitman Medical)

De Roo, M., Walravens, M. and Dequeker, J. (1978). Sacro-iliac disease and low backache in women. *Lancet*, **2**, 942

Golding, D.N. (1982). Some problems of backache in women. In Wright, V. (ed.). *Topical Reviews in Rheumatic Disorders*, pp. 203–218. (Bristol: Wright PSG)

Stoddard, A. (1981). *The Back – Relief from Pain. 3rd Edn.*(London: Martin Dunitz)

9
The Home Treatment of Backache

1. IMMEDIATE TREATMENT OF THE ACUTE ATTACK

When it occurs at home an acute attack of back pain can be quite alarming, both to the patient and his family. It sometimes seems to be precipitated by quite a minor event (or even a 'non-event', such as shaving). There is sudden excruciating pain which may radiate to the buttock or down the leg. Radiation of pain does not necessarily imply a 'slipped disc', as this can be simply referred pain and is usually not due to pressure on a lumbar nerve root.

The following procedure is a guide to emergency treatment of acute low back pain with or without sciatica.

(1)   The patient should lie on a firm surface with not more than one pillow. He should adopt the most comfortable position, which is not necessarily flat on his back – often he is most comfortable lying on his side with the knees bent up.

(2)   Two or three analgesic tablets preferably containing codeine are given (e.g. Panadeine Co. or Codeine Co.). Should these not be available, paracetamol or aspirin may be helpful. For some patients the beneficial effect will be enhanced by a double whisky!

(3)   Heat is applied to the lumbar spine by means of a covered hot-water bottle or heat pad. Alternatively, the patient may find cold compresses or an ice-pack more effective.

(4)   Should there not be relief of pain within 2–3 hours the family

doctor may be called. A stronger analgesic (such as dihydro-codeine (DF 118) or buprenorphine), or perhaps an intra-muscular injection of diazepam or pentazocine, or if necessary pethidine, may be required (see Chapter 3). The physician may advise further prolonged complete bed rest or alternatively may decide to manipulate the spine.

(5)   In severe or persisting pain, the consultant rheumatologist or orthopaedic surgeon may be called on a domiciliary visit and in certain cases admission to hospital may be advised.

(6)   Should the pain settle within a few hours or perhaps days the patient is gradually allowed to sit up, stand and then walk a few steps. At this stage physiotherapy is often helpful and ideally should be immediately available at the local hospital where there should be open access to physiotherapy by general practitioners (see Chapter 5).

(7)   If the acute attack subsides but there is residual pain, a consult-ation with the rheumatologist or orthopaedic surgeon may be advised.

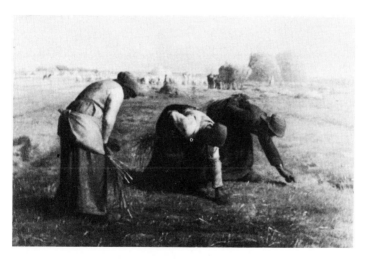

Figure 35 *Les Glaneuses*, by Millet (Louvre). The peasants demonstrate the incorrect way to bend and pick up objects from the ground

2.   HOME EXERCISES AND BACK DISCIPLINE

By *back discipline* is meant the correct way of using the back in the course of everyday activities. The patient may be told he has a 'weakness' or 'weak spot' in his back (be it a 'slipped disc', joint derangement or osteoarthritis) and that he must respect this 'spot' by observing correct back discipline, so avoiding future trouble. For example, there are correct and incorrect ways of bending and lifting (see Figures 35 and 36).

It is useful to provide the patient with a 'handout' depicting *back discipline and exercises* which shows correct and incorrect ways of stooping, kneeling and sitting. An example is given at the end of this chapter. More detailed information, including excellent illustrations, can be found in *The Back – Relief from Pain* by A. Stoddard – a book written for patients.

However the acute attack is treated, afterwards the physician or physiotherapist should give the patient a simple programme of prophylactic exercises to be done regularly at home. The following is a simple regime of back *extension exercises* (see Figure 23).

Patient handout: back exercises

Exercising should *not* be done during acute, painful back pain but when the pain is subsiding and especially afterwards, to try to prevent future attacks. Exercises should be done regularly (e.g. two or three times daily) on a firm surface (no pillows allowed). They should *not* be painful: *avoid any painful exercise, to the others*. Start gently, gradually increase the exercises day by day.

Here are *four basic back extension exercises:* two on the back, two on the stomach.

1. Lie on back, bend knees, lift bottom, hold 1 second, slowly lower bottom. Repeat.

2. Lie on back, lift each leg in turn, straighten leg up as far as possible, hold 1 second, slowly lower. Repeat.

3. Turn on stomach. Lift each leg in turn (with the knee straight) as far as possible, hold 1 second, slowly lower. Repeat.

4. Still on stomach, clasp hands behind head, arch back as much as possible, hold 5 seconds, relax slowly, rest for 5 seconds. Repeat.

Repeat each exercise until tiring, then go on to the next exercise. Try and increase the duration of each exercise each time you do back exercises.

A simple exercise for toning up the *abdominal muscles* is to lie supine and move the legs as if riding a bicycle, starting with the legs bent well up and then moving the feet further away.

A simple *'postural exercise'* (i.e. to improve the posture) which can be

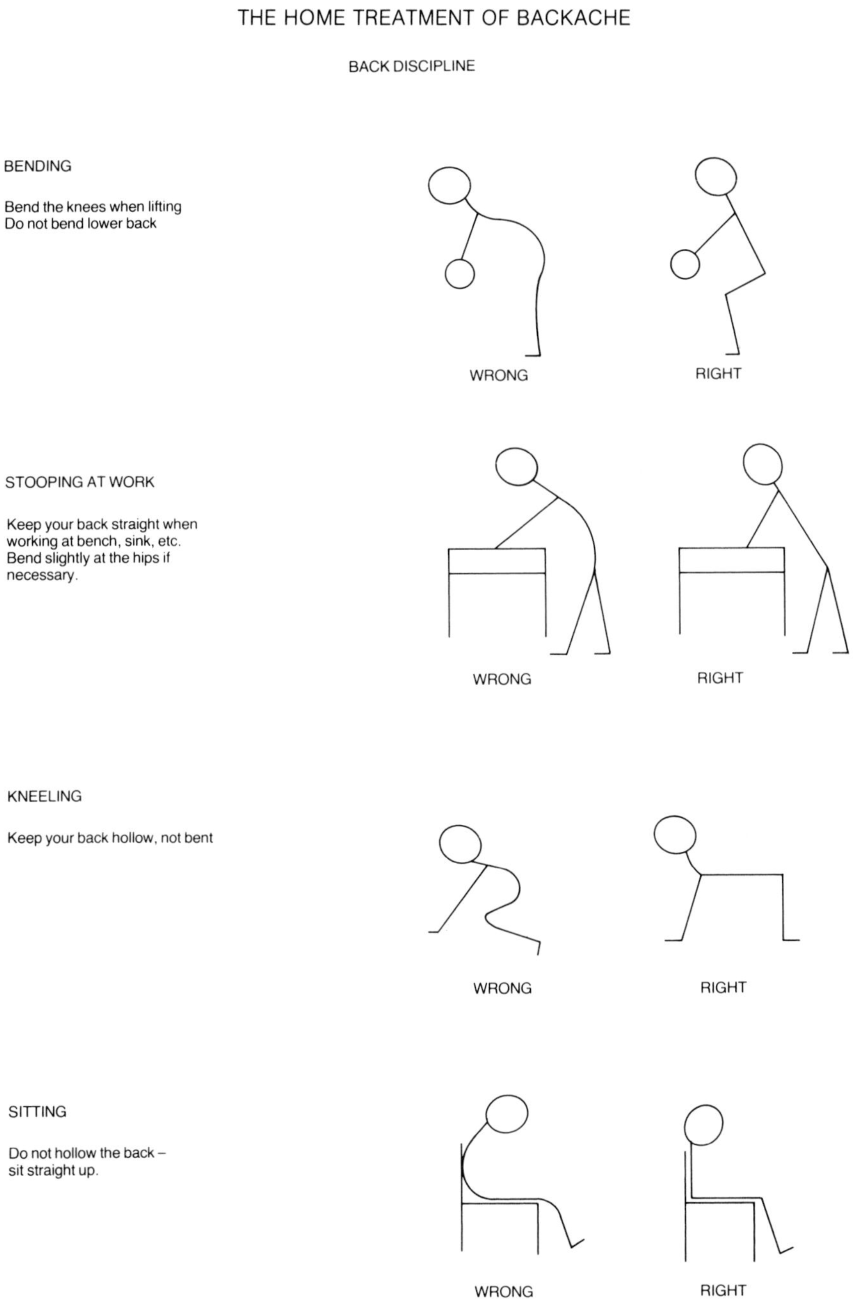

BACK DISCIPLINE

BENDING

Bend the knees when lifting
Do not bend lower back

WRONG   RIGHT

STOOPING AT WORK

Keep your back straight when
working at bench, sink, etc.
Bend slightly at the hips if
necessary.

WRONG   RIGHT

KNEELING

Keep your back hollow, not bent

WRONG   RIGHT

SITTING

Do not hollow the back –
sit straight up.

WRONG   RIGHT

Figure 36 A 'handout' for back discipline

done at home is 'standing tall' – in doing this the abdomen flattens,
the lumbar spine straightens and the buttock muscle contracts.

SUMMARY OF HOME TREATMENT

The patient should:

(1) Observe back discipline in bending, stooping, kneeling and sitting.

(2) Carry out regular simple home exercises.

(3) Sit correctly, with adequate back support.

(4) Use lumbar pillows for badly-designed seats, especially in cars.

Reference

Stoddard, A. (1981). *The Back – Relief from Pain*. 3rd Edn. (London: Martin Dunitz)

10
Conservative Treatment in Hospital

1. INDICATIONS FOR HOSPITAL TREATMENT

In previous chapters reference has been made to the indications for admission of patients suffering from backache to hospital. They can be summarized as follows:

(1) *Acute low back pain* which has failed to respond to a few days' home bed rest and/or one or two manipulations or a course of physiotherapy. Admission is particularly indicated if sciatica, indicating lateral disc prolapse, develops during this period. Admission may also be required if the nursing facilities at home are so poor that complete bed rest is impossible.

(2) *Acute sciatica* (with or without central or eccentric low back pain), which has failed to respond to adequate bed rest at home and perhaps a course of intermittent lumbar traction in the physiotherapy department, and where relevant (see Chapter 8) a therapeutic epidural injection has been tried.

(3) *Chronic sciatic pain* (due to longstanding disc prolapse, adhesion of lumbar nerve roots following previous disc surgery or severe chronic osteoarthritis of the lumbar spine) unresponsive to out-patient treatment.

(4) *Organic pathology* suspected, particularly neoplastic conditions, when hospitalization is preferred to facilitate intensive investigation as well as pain-relief.

Prolonged (more than 3 weeks) treatment in hospital (or in bed at home) is *not* indicated for mechanical lesions of the spinal joints or discs, where mobilization of the affected segment rather than rest is required.

Admission to hospital is of course required for spinal *surgery*. Most surgeons require a trial period of bed rest with traction in hospital before embarking upon surgical treatment (see Chapter 11).

2. CONSERVATIVE TREATMENT OF LUMBAR DISC LESIONS

The patient often has severe back pain and sciatica on admission. On the first day he or she is put to *bed in the most comfortable position* – usually (though not always) flat on his or her back, being allowed only one pillow. The mattress should be on a firm base (see also Chapter 3) but it is a myth that *all* patients with backache like a 'hard bed' – various degrees of firmness should be tried, the aim being to achieve maximum comfort in bed (see also chapter 8, section 3).

Adequate analgesics are prescribed 'around the clock'. If paracetamol 1 g 4-hourly provides insufficient analgesia, Panadeine Co. may be substituted. Strong analgesics such as dihydrocodeine or buprenorphine are prescribed on request, for example, 6-hourly p.r.n. A *muscle relaxant* such as diazepam can help 'break' the severe initial pain, especially if there is a big anxiety component, and small doses are given thereafter. At night, a tranquillizer or temazepam is prescribed. If there is significant depression an antidepressive drug such as amitriptyline 25–75 mg should be prescribed.

On the day after admission the patient has become more 'settled' and relaxed. *Continuous pelvic traction* (see chapter 4, section 7) is then applied, unless there is still severe muscle rigidity when the dose of diazepam should be progressively increased until the spasm is adequately controlled. Only then will continuous traction have its desired effect – besides producing distraction of the spine, traction has the additional advantage of keeping the patient still; complete rest is still the most important factor in treating acute disc lesions. A pelvic harness is fitted and approximately 20 kg weight is applied, using pulleys at the end of the bed. The foot of the bed is usually raised 15–30 cm (see Figure 26). Traction should be removed at night if it disturbs sleep – painful or uncomfortable traction is deleterious rather than helpful. It may also be removed for 30 minutes once or twice daily to give the patient a 'rest'; during these periods some patients appreciate a pillow under the knees. Progress is monitored by decrease in leg pain and improvement in straight-leg-raising and occasionally there is improvement in deep reflexes. Improvement may occur within

1 or 2 weeks when traction can be progressively removed for an hour, 2 hours and then several hours every day, the patient being allowed to sit on the edge of the bed, then sit up in a chair for half an hour twice-daily, then walk slowly to the toilet. At this point *gentle extension exercises* are introduced and the patient is *gradually mobilized*, being allowed to walk down the corridor and (weather permitting) out in the garden. Before discharge home he or she is warned to 'back pedal' a little and take it easy for at least another week, as it is only too easy to suddenly overdo matters on returning home. It is often advisable to supply a *temporary light lumbar support* to be worn for the first few weeks after discharge, and this is especially required if return to manual work is to be allowed within the near future so that some prophylactic support for the back is provided.

3. THE NON-RESOLVING DISC

If after 2 or at the most 3 weeks' bed rest and traction in hospital sciatic pain persists and straight-leg-raising fails to improve substantially, it is advisable to arrange a *myelogram* to decide on the severity of the prolapse (or prolapses) and the extent of nerve root involvement with reference to possible surgical treatment. Myelograms using a non-irritant water-soluble opaque medium which is later absorbed from the subarachnoid space (known as radiculograms) will also demonstrate an alternative space-occupying lesion (such as a tumour) which could be responsible for the symptoms. Unfortunately, for a day or two after radiculography headache and nausea and occasionally more troublesome neurotoxic side-effects are not uncommon, but not the more serious after-effects common after myelography. Additional evidence of the site or sites of prolapse is provided by electromyographic studies on the leg muscles which demonstrate denervation of segmental muscle groups corresponding to the root supply. (Other recently-introduced techniques for demonstrating disc prolapse are epidurography, ascending lumbar venography and discography. These are not in general use – for a description of these techniques the reader is referred to Jayson's *The Lumbar Spine and Back Pain*).

Should symptoms persist but the disc prolapse is 'small' (as shown by pain of no great severity, absence of motor weakness and only slight or moderate limitation of straight-leg-raising) a *caudal epidural injection* may be tried as a possible alternative to surgery (see Chapter 8). A single epidural injection may be tried first, or a continuous lumbar epidural using a catheter can sometimes be effective when a caudal epidural fails; pain decreases or disappears within a few days and straight-leg-raising increases, when the patient may be mobilized quite quickly and return home within a day or two. (Epidural injections are also useful for outpatient treatment – see Chapter 8.)

Large disc prolapses not responding to bed rest with traction in hospital, and also smaller prolapses not responding to bed rest and/or epidural injections, will probably require *surgery* (see Chapter 11).

SUMMARY: CONSERVATIVE TREATMENT IN HOSPITAL

(1)   The indications for hospital treatment of backache and sciatica are summarized at the beginning of this chapter.

(2)   Bed rest with analgesics, relaxants, night sedatives and anti-depressive drugs if required is instituted from the first day.

(3)   Continuous pelvic traction is applied from the day after admission for a period varying from 1 to 3 weeks, when traction is progressively removed and mobilization started.

(4)   Myelography is indicated where symptoms fail to improve with bed rest and traction. Electromyelograms may also help to locate the levels of the disc lesion or lesions.

(5)   Caudal epidural injections may accelerate recovery in the case of small disc prolapses.

(6)   Surgical treatment may be indicated for disc lesions which fail to resolve with the above treatment.

Reference

Jayson, M. (ed.). (1980). *The Lumbar Spine and Back Pain*. 2nd Edn. (London: Pitman Medical)

11
The Place of Surgery in Back Pain and Sciatica

1. SURGERY FOR LUMBAR DISC PROTRUSIONS

Although the great majority of backache and sciatica is amenable to conservative treatment, nevertheless surgery has an important role in the management of a number of cases of prolapsed intervertebral disc (PID) in the lumbar spine. Disc surgery is not to be undertaken lightly, but only when certain well-defined criteria for operation are satisfied. Even in the best hands surgery is not uniformly successful: about 10–20% do not receive benefit and the exact figure depends on the strictness with which the surgeon selects his cases and his experience with disc surgery. Again, even where the initial result is satisfactory about 50% patients have minor residual symptoms and the recurrence rate of major symptoms may be as high as 15%. Such recurrences, whether at the same disc level or a fresh one, are difficult to treat by conservative means and second operations are hazardous, carrying a success rate below 50%. It may not be wise to return a patient to heavy manual work after surgery because of this risk. It is no doubt significant that, before the advent of disc surgery, the majority of patients recovered spontaneously given time. Although natural recovery often takes 6–18 months it is often felt that if the pain is bearable it may be better to wait because, though surgery offers a more rapid result, if there is a recurrence afterwards the outlook is worse.

Apart from the cauda equina syndrome or a progressive root palsy there is no particular symptom or physical sign that demands surgery;

for example, neurological features such as numbness or moderate muscle weakness can be usually ignored as they will recover in time, and so it follows that in the vast majority of cases it is only the severity of pain that causes the patient and the doctor to look to surgery for an answer. The doctor has to take an objective view in asking himself 'are there definite indications that surgery will relieve this patient?' If not, he must be firm and refuse to refer the patient – there is no place for exploratory operations on the spine. In practice this is often difficult: for example, where a young woman with a low pain threshold has had unrelenting, demoralizing sciatica for many months there is great pressure from the patient, relatives and often the family doctor for action. Where there is a neurotic trait or a claim for compensation outstanding it is especially important to be sure that there are suitable objective indications for surgery. The usual indications have been outlined by Naylor (1977). (See below.)

The basic surgical procedure for lumbar disc lesions is *laminectomy*,

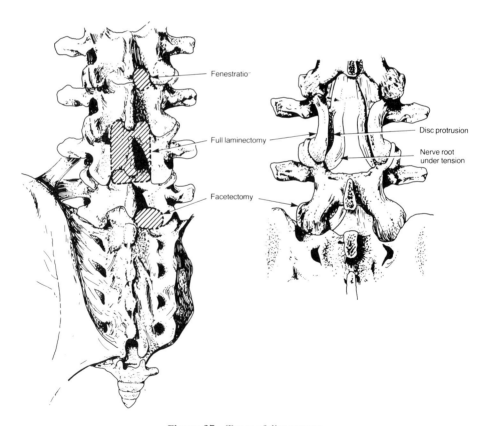

Figure 37 Types of disc surgery

98

but this generic term covers several different techniques. Most surgeons start with an interlaminar approach where the yellow ligament is excised on one side and then bone nibbled away from the adjacent laminae until a small gap is made through which the nerve root and the disc protrusion can be visualized (often called fenestration). If this fails to give adequate exposure of the offending disc or discs then the surgeon may proceed to remove the whole laminae and spinous process at one level, when the disc can be explored from both sides. It is important to ensure that the nerve root is free and under no tension as far as the exit foramen; if the root is compressed in the lateral recess of the spinal canal between the facet-joint and an osteophyte at the level of the disc, it is necessary to remove part of the facet-joint (facetectomy) to release the nerve. (Figure 37).

After a successful operation the patient often gets immediate relief of sciatic pain. Usually he is allowed up after 3 days, back exercises are commenced by the seventh day and he goes home after 14 days. The average patient can return to work after 6 weeks, although he may still have some low back pain and aching in the leg from time to time. There is no evidence that keeping the patient off work for longer produces a better final result and indeed this can be counter-productive in demoralizing the patient; it is better to warn him to expect some residual symptoms, and to reassure him that it is safe to start work.

Failure of operative treatment to relieve symptoms can become apparent in two ways: there may be no relief right from the start, or there may be a symptom-free interval followed by return of symptoms. Immediate failure to relieve symptoms may be due to one of the following:

(1) removal of the wrong disc,
(2) no disc protrusion found at operation
(3) incomplete freeing of the nerve root in the lateral recess of the spinal canal.

An interval of relief lasting a number of weeks before pain returns may well be due to the period of enforced bed rest, the actual operating having been a failure. If the pain-free interval is longer than a few weeks but no more than 6 months, recurrence of pain may be due to *arachnoiditis*, a troublesome inflammation of the meninges with subsequent fibrosis. Postoperatively some degree of scar tissue in this area is inevitable, but why this gives rise to pain in a minority of patients and not in others is unknown. Unfortunately, the pain of arachnoiditis is intractable without satisfactory treatment. If the pain-free interval is greater than 6 months the most likely cause of return of pain is a further disc herniation, either at the same or at a new level.

The *indications for surgery for lumbar disc lesions* may be summarized as follows:

(1)   Cauda equina syndrome (see Chapter 3).

(2)   Progressive root palsy, or a very recent complete root palsy. When a root palsy becomes complete there may be cessation of pain, making it difficult to decide whether surgery should go ahead. If the palsy is very recent there is some chance of recovery of useful motor power following surgery, but if an interval has elapsed there is no point in decompressing the nerve.

(3)   Persistent severe and unacceptable sciatic pain, the following being present:
(a) definite neurological deficit (e.g. an absent reflex)
(b) positive tension signs (straight-leg-raising or femoral nerve stretch)
(c) positive radiculogram, showing one or more disc prolapses.

With these provisions in mind two groups of patients may require surgery for persistent sciatica – those suffering from either:

(1)   Severe acute sciatica not resolving with adequate (hospital) conservative treatment over a period of 3–6 weeks, or

(2)   chronic sciatica, taking the form of either recurrent disabling attacks (for example, 4 weeks off work each year) or permanent pain.

In the past some surgeons carried out simultaneous fusion of the joints, particularly if there was any indication of instability. Lumbar fusion has largely fallen out of favour as there is little evidence that it leads to a better result, and it increases the severity and risk of the operation and makes access to the spinal canal impossible should there be further root pressure in the future.

2. SURGERY FOR SPONDYLOLISTHESIS

Spondylolisthesis (forward slip of one vertebra on the vertebra below – see Chapter 1.2) may be due to a bilateral defect in the pars interarticularis or degenerative changes in the disc joint leading to laxity of the annulus fibrosis and overriding of the facets. In general, defects in the pars lead to a much greater degree of 'slip' than does disc degeneration. Disc degeneration may alternatively lead to a backward slip of one vertebra on the other, known as *retrospondylolisthesis*. Most patients with back pain due to spondylolisthesis or retrolisthesis can receive adequate relief from a firm lumbar support and sensible reduction of heavy work. However, a significant number suffer intractable backache or sciatica and surgery has to be considered.

Where backache is the predominant symptom in spondylolisthesis, surgical fusion is considered:

(1)   In young patients with a bilateral defect of the pars interarticularis and marked backache preventing them leading an active life.

(2)   In middle-aged patients with severe backache which is not controlled by a corset but is completely relieved by lying down. There must be considerable instability, demonstrable radiographically. Unfortunately, there is a risk that even after successful fusion and a number of years of relief symptoms may recommence as extra strain falls on the segment above the fusion.

(Fusion is rarely advised for elderly patients with spondylolisthesis, who must usually rely on a corset and analgesics.)

Where sciatica is the prominent symptom, this may be due to:

(1)   The development of a disc prolapse at the unstable joint, when laminectomy alone is usually performed though in young active patients fusion may also be necessary.

(2)   In the older age group, where degenerative changes are marked (osteophytosis of the vertebral margins and around the facet-joints) sciatica may be due to bony impingement on a nerve root, when releasing tension on the nerve root by removal of part of the facet-joint and adjacent lamina gives a satisfactory result. (One might expect this type of operation to increase the vertebral instability and lead to further 'slip', but this is not so in practice – there is no increase in backache and the relief of the nerve pain allows much improvement in standing and walking.)

3.   SURGERY FOR SPINAL STENOSIS

This important cause of back pain, sciatica and often neurogenic claudication has been mentioned in Chapter 1.2, where it is pointed out that degenerative changes in the disc and facet joints precipitate symptoms in an already narrow trefoil canal, often at L_5 or S_1. Patients have a history of low back pain, then usually bilateral leg pain and paraesthesiae which often appear as neurogenic (as opposed to vascular) claudication. Flexing the spine for 5–10 minutes relieves symptoms by increasing the size of the spinal canal so that, unlike vascular claudication, exercise on the static bicycle in the physiotherapy department does not bring on pain, as the back is flexed while cycling. Examination may reveal little – reasonable back movements and straight-leg-raising, possibly a reduced ankle-jerk. Investigations include measurement of the spinal canal by the radiologist, and myelography. CAT scans (computerized axial tomography) may find a use in showing the shapes and sizes of the canal, and ultrasound be used to measure the sagittal diameter of the canal.

Lumbar traction or a caudal epidural injection is often effective in mild neurogenic claudication due to spinal stenosis. Otherwise surgery is required (see Gabris, 1980). This often gives satisfying results, but is not invariably effective. The canal is decompressed by removing the laminae at several levels, together with partial resection of the facet-joints to 'unroof' the lateral recesses. Afterwards patients are usually mobilized for a few days and given a lumbar corset.

SUMMARY

The principal operations for backache and sciatica are as follows.

(1) Laminectomy – for relief of persisting sciatica due to intervertebral disc prolapse.

(2) Lumbar fusion – the main indication is spondylolisthesis with defect in the pars interarticularis in a young person. May be considered in middle-aged patients with intractable backache and demonstrable vertebral instability and complete relief on lying down.

(3) Decompression of spinal canal – for elderly patients with spinal stenosis causing neurogenic claudication not responding to conservative treatment.

References

Gabris, S. (1980). *J. Bone J. Surg.*, **62A**, 308
Naylor, A. (1977). *Br. Med. J.*, **1**, 567

Index